CW00506272

<u>IN CASE YOU LOSE THIS BOOK:</u>

Hello!

This book is so incredibly important to me.

If you've found it, that means I've gone and bloody lost it.

So, pretty please, with a cherry on top, contact me using the details below, so I can make arrangements to retrieve it.

Thank you so much!

Name...

Email..

Phone...

praise for *the off the rocks journal*

'In *The Off The Rocks Journal*, Jennie Nelson brings together all of the most effective self-help tools for tackling compulsive and addictive behaviours in one simple, cohesive and practical system. I've been waiting for a book like this for years. It is the perfect companion for anyone seriously committed to positive and lasting change.'
Pauline Brumwell, Psychotherapeutic Counsellor and Hypnotherapist.

'*The Off The Rocks Journal* is a brilliant resource, particularly for people who want to take control of compulsive behaviours and are looking for practical tools to help them. In this book, motivation and inspiration are combined with credible techniques that have been proven to work – enabling people to track their development and see the progress they are making. This innovative journal goes beyond simply providing advice and guidance; it can become an integral part of the process of recovery and change.'
Russell Kelsey, GP and Author of *Patient Safety: Investigating and Reporting Serious Clinical Incidents*.

'*The Off The Rocks Journal* would be an amazing addition to anyone seeking to improve their life. I think tracking, cataloguing and diarising things can make such a monumental difference. It's all about linking up our moods with what we put into, and do, to our bodies, and seeing the patterns. Honesty, accountability and journaling can have such a dramatic effect on our lifestyle choices, and that is why this book is a life-changer.'
Catherine Gray, author of *The Unexpected Joy of Being Sober* and *The Unexpected Joy of Being Single*.

'With the NHS at breaking point it is clear that we need to change something. Prescribing pills does little to change lives. People inevitably go home with medication only to live the same way that got them into trouble in the first place, causing them to go back to their doctor within a few months with exactly the same symptoms and problems. I love *The Off The Rocks Journal* because it arms people with the tools they need to get themselves well. It teaches people how to mindfully address the things that are holding them back, rather than trying to mask symptoms with medications or other vices. It's a fantastic mix of nutrition, exercise, psychology and spirituality, all written in an engaging way by someone who clearly knows what they are talking about. Jennie writes from the heart and, through intelligent use of science and her own experience, has put together something truly special.'
Dr Jack Darby, GP and Qualified Personal Trainer.

'Journaling is a brilliant idea for keeping on track; I think Jennie has a great concept with *The Off The Rocks Journal*. It will be genuinely helpful for people. There are several clinical studies that prove a food diary is the best way to stay healthy.'

Kate Faithful-Williams, Certified Health Coach writer and author of *The Feelgood Plan - Happier, Healthier and Slimmer in 15 Minutes a Day.*

'Jennie has created an impressive journal that allows its reader to effectively monitor the fundamental basics of any healthy lifestyle. As a personal trainer I have managed hundreds of clients, many of them professional athletes, so I'm continuously reminded about the importance of tracking progress. I always advise anyone who wants to improve their health to start by keeping an accurate food diary and a record of their exercise routine. Without this, they are simply guessing, and at times of plateaus and back-sliding, it's difficult to see how they are going off track. *The Off The Rocks Journal* successfully manages to make doing these vitally important things easy, effective, and enjoyable.'

Sam Johnstone, Certified Personal Trainer and founder of *Sam Johnstone Coaching.*

'Tracking, logging, monitoring - whatever you prefer to call it, is always going to be a game-changer for anyone looking, not only to improve their health, but to seek a new-found quality of life. It gives us new evidence and highlights the ramifications of old habits that can keep us hostage. As a personal trainer I understand the importance and benefits of logging: "If you log, you learn!" It helps give vision and purpose in times of difficulty. Change is not an act but a habit. Typically what we *think* we do, and what we *actually* do, are two different things. Tracking our progress helps us to become more mindful; restoring balance to our lifestyles, helping us to become more accountable and open to change. In *The Off The Rocks Journal*, Jennie is giving us the tools to help make that happen in a very simple, achievable way. Remember: "If you're not assessing you're guessing!" Happy journaling.'

Richard J Clark. Certified Health & Fitness Coach and founder of *365 Function.*

<u>THIS BOOK IS DEDICATED TO:</u>

My glorious fellow flounderers who've yet to see: you get to save yourself!

This is from me to you, with nothing but love, love, love.

Jen xo

contents

the jennie nelson story

If you're anything like me, it doesn't take much to throw you off track. I'm a million times better than I used to be, but that's mostly because I used to be absolutely ridiculous. I wouldn't so much get thrown off track, as I would wilfully wander off, blaming everything but myself for the course that my life was taking. In the past, a bad day could last anything up to six months and during that time I'd change just about everything except my perspective.

I first created the concept for this book a few years ago when I recognised that my life was in need of a massive overhaul. I was working hard and partying harder. I was a breakfast show radio presenter at the time and my rollercoaster lifestyle was seriously catching up with me.

My typical work day started at 4am and I was live on air with my co-host from 6-9am every week-day. I also hosted my own live bands show on Sunday afternoons and I'd often be asked to work for the radio station on Saturdays too. Whether it was an outside broadcast, presenting big, boozy awards ceremonies or being out and about doing meet and greets with our listeners; I was always busy. I was always knackered. I was always playing catch up.

I'd chug endless cups of strong sugary tea and cans of full fat coke during the day and neck dangerous amounts of alcohol most nights. I was constantly sleep-deprived and my eating habits were all over the place. Back then I was a chain smoking, caffeine glugging, junk food scoffing, wine swilling, work addicted, party animal. My friends couldn't keep up with me, my family were worried about me and I drove my boyfriends bonkers.

I was living my life in a deeply unhealthy way. I'd become heavily reliant on all the wrong things. I'd come to depend on external props to support me: career, caffeine, cigarettes, alcohol, fast food, boyfriends. This sort of behaviour isn't uncommon. We all struggle with bad habits and sab-otage ourselves in different ways to varying degrees, and we each reach our limits at different points too. Once I'd reached my lowest ebb I knew I had to make some big changes and that was how I came to write this book.

I didn't fully realise it at the time but my bad habits were all intertwined and tangled up. One be-haviour would impact on another and so it never really worked whenever I tried to address just one problem area. Which I'd often try to do, thinking that if I fixed one problem, everything else would magically fall into place. But it doesn't work that way. You know when you gently pull at a loose thread and you inadvertently yank down the whole hem? It felt like that. I was unravelling. Even when I was trying my hardest to make things better. I felt like I'd gotten into such a muddle that I needed a fundamental shake up in every area of my life in order to properly sort myself out.

I needed a radical re-evaluation and I needed a way to document my progress and keep me motivated. So I went back to basics, stripping away everything that wasn't healthy or necessary. I decided to ditch the drink completely. Alcohol had become an obvious unhealthy coping mechanism for me by then. I would turn to it for everything and found it hard to imagine a life without it. I knew I'd become over-reliant on it and that I was using it to cope with other problems. When I was anxious, I'd drink. When I felt down, I'd drink. When I felt happy, I'd drink. It was my go-to quick fix but it had started exacerbating more problems than it solved. It had to go, possibly forever, certainly for a while.

Going teetotal meant that I could address all of my other problems with far better clarity. It took a lot of getting used to and was hard at first, but I went stone-cold sober for nearly five years in the end and was prepared to never drink alcohol again if that's what it took. I started lifting weights at the gym five times a week on average. I ate clean, healthy wholefoods, adopting a 99% plant based diet. I learnt how to cook properly from scratch. I took up new hobbies. I saw a qualified therapist every week. I joined support groups and forums. I read hundreds of recommended books and watched loads of acclaimed documentaries. I listened to countless podcasts. I researched every area of my life that I had an issue with, and did all the suggested work. I changed the way I related to people. I switched jobs. I moved house. I helped others. I went on courses. I travelled. I journaled. I recorded my progress. I documented what worked for me and what didn't. I started a daily meditation practice. I got back into yoga. I exercised extreme self-discipline and radical self-care. I was completely honest with myself and others. I addressed my anxiety and depression. I lovingly detached from people, places and things that made me feel wobbly. I cultivated patience. I made mistakes. I learnt from my mistakes. I didn't give up. I took full accountability for my own life and I pursued my long-term health and happiness with the same passion that I'd once chased short-lived hedonism. At times it was tough, really, really rough, but oh my gosh, it was so incredibly worth it.

During that time I came up with a scrappy little prototype for the book you're holding in your hands right now - and it worked. It worked like an absolute charm! My healthy lifestyle overhaul didn't happen overnight, it wasn't easy and it wasn't without considerable trial and error. Some aspects of my life took longer to address than others because some bad habits were more entrenched. But genuine, authentic, freedom from my old wounded ways was mine and it's been mine every second of every day ever since - with the help of this book.

We all struggle with things from time to time and we've all experienced trauma to one degree or another. It's all part of the sometimes marvellous, sometimes messy business of being alive. Unfortunately, the ways in which we cope with our discomfort aren't always the healthiest. They can often harm and hurt us all the more. Routinely turning to greasy takeaways or bingeing on booze might suppress sadness in the short term, but in the long run that sort of behaviour tends to make matters worse. Especially if those behaviours become established coping strategies and something we start to compulsively depend on. It's been said that addiction is a symptom of untreated pain and that any substance or behaviour a person is addicted to, is an indication of an underlying problem. To become healthier and happier, our underlying problems must be addressed alongside whatever substance abuse or dysfunctional behaviour we've become reliant on. Addiction isn't a yes or no issue, it's a spectrum condition and we're all on the scale somewhere for one thing or another. But I think we have more control over our compulsions than we're often led to believe and we owe it to ourselves to get unshackled without feeling the shame that's so often attached to the issue of addiction. There's nothing to feel ashamed about and we don't have to hit a catastrophic rock bottom before we realise there's a happier way to live.

Your happiness, just like mine, is there for the taking, anytime you want to go after it, it just takes time, effort, patience and the right tools. It is hard work but it *is* worth it. *You* are worth it, you truly are. And anyway, doing the work is a lot easier than living a half-life that you're miserable in and too frightened to let go of.

I hope that this book helps you to understand yourself a bit better. I hope it inspires you and motivates you and reminds you that you alone are responsible for your own life, nobody else. You have enormous power to contribute to either your happiness or your despair and the choice is always yours. Everything you need to live your happiest, most beautiful life, is already inside you. It's just that sometimes we forget how much we're capable of and we need a little help to remember. So this is your gentle, loving reminder: go for it!

Love, Jen xo

<u>what this book can do for you</u>

'On the rocks' is a well-worn phrase that means: experiencing difficulties and likely to fail. Synonyms: in difficulty, in trouble, breaking down.

Well, hey! Welcome to The *Off* The Rocks Journal - this book will help to guide you *away* from difficulties, troubles and breakdowns and towards a big, bright, lovely life that you're happy and proud to live.

If you feel like you're on the rocks in any way, you're in good company. Half of us are overweight. Most marriages end in divorce and more people than ever before are depressed, anxious and addicted to something that desensitises them to their discomfort. This book, if you invest in it, will help you to get off the rocks and back on track.

If you feel like something is holding you back from living the happiest life of your wildest dreams, The Off The Rocks Journal can help you to work out what it is and what you can do about it.

Maybe you drink too much and can't seem to moderate?
Maybe you comfort eat too often or smoke even though you'd rather stop?
Perhaps you're depending on sleeping pills and caffeine because you're unable to sleep at night or get going in the morning?
Maybe your relationships are suffering and your health is spiralling, you're overstressed and underwhelmed and can't quite seem to get back on top of things?

If any of that sounds familiar - this book is made for you.

We all know that good health - physical, mental and emotional - is absolutely imperative to living a happy life. It's the foundation on which a happy life is built. Yet so many of us are unintentionally and continuously sabotaging ourselves in all manner of ways. Seeking happiness in things that disrupt our health and actively cause *un*happiness. Things like junk food, late nights and booze binges. Routinely choosing to slump on the sofa instead of stretching our legs outside in the fresh air. Why do we do this to ourselves? How does all this short-term gratification impact on us in the long-term? How do we find the motivation to make healthier lasting changes?

The Off The Rocks Journal is designed to help you make sense of your life so that you can be free to make the choices that support your goals. It is the ultimate interactive health journal. There is nothing else quite like it.

The benefits of keeping even an ordinary journal are well known, but the benefits of using The Off The Rocks Journal are unparalleled. This is because it incorporates everything you need to keep track of in order to live your healthiest life: diet, exercise, what we do, how we feel, what we worry about and how we cope with our worries - these are all things that we need to pay consistent mindful attention to, but it's often hard to know where to start. Our lives are so busy. Our to-do lists are so long and our time is so short. This book brilliantly simplifies our over-complicated lifestyles.

First things first: Stop. Just stop. Right now. Slow down. Take a moment and breathe.

Everything you need is already within your grasp, I promise you. You just need to realise your own boundless potential. You can overcome anything that you set your mind to. You just need the right tools to help you do it - and now you do.

The Off The Rocks Journal can help you to completely transform your life. You can start any time you like and address any type of problem area. Whatever your personal goals, whatever your individual struggles, whatever it is that you want to take control of in your life, this book can help you to achieve, overcome and accomplish.

The Off The Rocks Journal runs for twelve consecutive months on a perpetual basis, meaning that you can start using it any time you like and it will last you for a whole year. Imagine how different your life could look just one year from now. You don't have to wait for the new year. You don't have to wait for your next birthday. You don't have to wait for a rock bottom. You don't have to wait another minute.

Buy this book, pour yourself into it, and start living the best days of your life from this moment on.

how it works

The Off The Rocks Journal is divided into twelve sections - one for every month of the year. You can start this journal at any time, just write the date at the top of each journal page. Each of the twelve sections starts with a short lifestyle essay. These punchy pieces are all chock-a-block with current, impartial, healthy-living content. They cover all of the fundamental areas of any healthy lifestyle. Use them to help guide and motivate you as you work your way through your journal.

Following each essay, there is a one-page monthly progress chart to fill out throughout the course of that particular month. Every day you will score yourself by marking a dot on each of the graphs in the relevant place - the dates of the month run across the top of the chart and the score line runs down the left hand side. The charts cover four of the most important areas of any healthy lifestyle: diet, exercise, life events and emotions. Each of the four charts are set out identically, but the way you gauge your self-judged score for each one is slightly different due to the nature of the thing being tracked. Don't worry, you'll soon get the hang of it once you start!

The scoring system, down the left hand side, runs from -3 to +3 with a bold line smack bang in the middle, which represents the baseline. The definition of a baseline is: a starting point used for comparisons. So think of the baseline for each of the charts as representing a middle-ground position, somewhere that's pretty good, but is also a great point to make further improvements from.

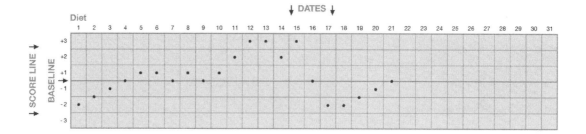

<u>how to gauge your score on the *diet* progress chart</u>

The diet chart includes everything you consume. Everything you put into your body contributes to your health in either a positive or a negative way and that includes every single thing you ingest; so when determining your overall score for your diet progress chart that day, include all foods, drinks, sweets, vitamins, dietary supplements, protein powders, caffeinated products, cigarettes, alcohol and any other drugs. If, for example, you are drinking more than one caffeinated drink per day and regularly consume alcohol, that will bring your score down. If you smoke, that will also contribute to lowering your score. If you're eating a lot of sugary foods and drinks or adding sugar to your tea or coffee, that too will bring your score down. As will regularly eating chocolate, processed foods or anything else that we know is unhealthy for us. On the other hand if you rarely eat unhealthy foods and are mostly going for lots of whole foods and grains, plenty of fruit, vegetables, seeds, herbal teas, juices and water then you'll be pushing your score up from the baseline and into the positive score numbers.

To give yourself a baseline score on the diet progress chart:
You'd need to be making fairly good nutritional choices at least 80% of the time.

<u>how to gauge your score on the *exercise* progress chart</u>

The exercise chart includes all the exercise you do. So whether you lift weights at the gym or just take your dog for a walk, it all counts. Obviously the more active you are, the better it is for your health, but every activity you do can be counted as part of your daily exercise quota if you put enough energy into it. Official NHS guidelines state that to stay healthy, adults ideally need to incorporate two types of physical activity into their routines; aerobic and strength exercises. Everything you do during any given day can contribute to your health in either a positive way or a negative way. So, for instance, if your job entails sitting at a desk all day and then you sit on your sofa all night, that would bring your exercise score down. Likewise, if you're regularly sitting in pubs at weekends, that will bring your score down too. If on the other hand you're always on the go, have hobbies that make you exert yourself and have a job that keeps you on your toes, that will all contribute to you getting more exercise that the minimum recommendation.

To give yourself a baseline score on the exercise progress chart:
You'd need to be doing the current recommended minimum of 30 minutes moderate aerobic activity per day. Moderate exercise is classed as any activity which raises your heart rate, makes you breathe faster and feel warmer.

how to gauge your score on the *life events* progress chart

A life event is any disruptive episode that occurs in your life - they can be big, or small, planned or unplanned, positive or negative. (For example, getting married, having a baby, having an argument with someone, having an operation or going on holiday.) Simply determine whether it was an overall positive life event or an overall negative life event, and to what extent, and then mark your dot in the appropriate place on your chart.

To give yourself a baseline score on the life events progress chart:

You'd need to feel that nothing much at all disrupted you in either a positive or negative way that day.

how to gauge your score on the *emotions* progress chart

Your emotions show how you feel and cope and our feelings are naturally changeable. We are all capable of many different emotions but they can generally be categorised into either pleasurable or displeasurable feelings. Either positive or negative. If you felt angry, upset or depressed you would score your emotions for that day *below* the baseline level, denoting the degree that you felt was accurate. If you felt happy or excited, you would score yourself somewhere *above* the baseline for that given emotion, depending on the degree of those feelings.

To give yourself a baseline score on the emotions progress chart:

You'd need to feel that you were on an even keel throughout the day. That you felt emotionally stable with no discernible variation in mood.

On the following page, there's a mock up of a progress chart, filled out in November 2018. As you can see, beneath the four main progress charts: **diet, exercise, life events** and **emotions**, is a spare one labelled **your choice**. This additional chart allows you to monitor anything else that you might want to. This example shows someone who's been monitoring their sleep quality. At the very bottom of the page, you'll see that there are two further mini charts to record any additional influences that you feel might be impacting on your health, either positively or negatively. For instance, you might want to monitor how your alcohol intake affects you. Many people drink to alleviate anxiety, not realising that it can contribute to anxiety at the same time that it masks it. Other additional influencers you could track are: anxiety, depression, cigarettes, caffeine, prescription drugs, vitamins, supplements, menstrual cycle, pornography use, gambling habits, fast food consumption. The list is non-exhaustive. If there is anything you feel particularly affected by, you can track it. In the example shown, this person has monitored their menstrual cycle and alcohol consumption. Simply label the mini chart, for example: 'alcohol', and mark an 'x' in the relevant date boxes on that mini chart whenever you consume any alcohol. Over time it will show on your charts how alcohol affects the other areas of your life whenever you drink it. Likewise, women's menstrual cycles can affect them to varying degrees in a multitude of ways. It's useful for everyone to understand how they are being influenced and to what extent.

The Off The Rocks progress charts are designed so that once you've filled them in, you can cut them out, without disrupting any other part of the book. *(Note the scissors icon down the left hand side of the example progress chart)*. Then you can tape them all together, in consecutive month order, and assess your lifestyle patterns over the course of several months at a quick glance.

You're then free to show this data to your doctor, therapist, personal trainer, nutritionalist, or anybody you like, to get objective advice, opinions and feedback on any patterns you might see. That way, your more detailed journal entry pages (to be explained further in just a moment) remain private. Still tucked away safely in your book.

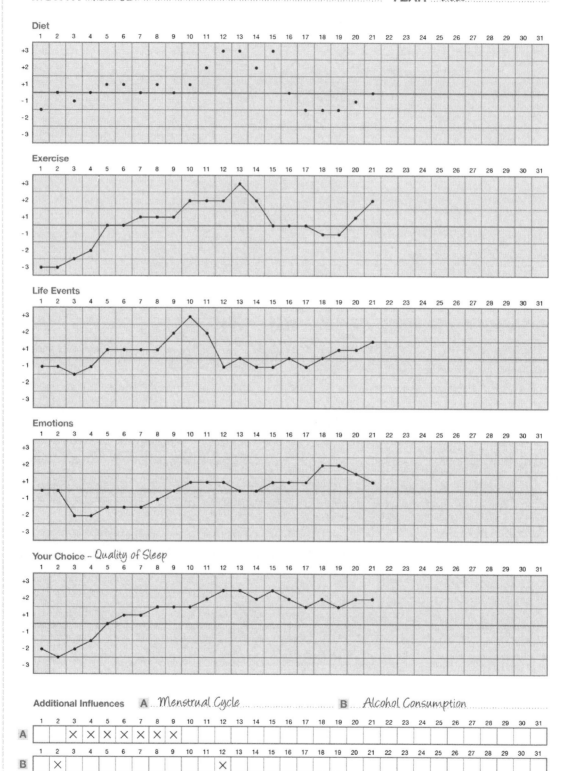

Diet

Exercise

Life Events

Emotions

Your Choice – *Quality of Sleep*

Additional Influences A *Menstrual Cycle*   B *Alcohol Consumption*

If your doctor, for example, asks what caused a particular spike, dip or sustained stable period on one aspect of your progress chart, you can refer to your private, more detailed journal entry pages on the corresponding days to find out exactly what was happening in your life at that time that might have contributed to, or caused, the variations seen on your charts. Perhaps you drank more alcohol than usual; which caused you to feel depressed afterwards or maybe your caffeine intake lessened; causing you to suffer withdrawal effects and suffer with anxiety symptoms. Maybe you picked up a sports injury, requiring enforced rest, which negatively affected your mood and your subsequent dietary choices. Whatever the influencing factors, you'll be able to accurately pinpoint them if there was anything you did differently to bring about the changes that occurred in your life at that time. (Please bear in mind that using the Off The Rocks Journal does not replace advice or supervision from your doctor.)

Filling out these charts every day will soon create a visual scale that will allow you to identify the presence, absence and/or severity of any problem areas. Join the dots as you go and day by day you will create a clear record of your individual behaviours and lifestyle choices, revealing any dips, peaks and periods of stability. Notice how your lifestyle choices directly impact on your overall health and happiness. At a glance you'll be able to see any trends or changes. You'll be able to fully appreciate how certain factors influence your behaviours and emotional states.

Finally, in each of the twelve sections of the journal, after the short essay and after the progress chart page, there are 31 identical journal entry pages - one for every day of that particular month. (Obviously, like the dates across the top of the progress charts, the shorter months of the year won't require all 31 spaces or pages. Just ignore the few spaces and pages that you don't use on those months.) The journal entry pages are are to be completed by you, by hand, one day at a time, sequentially, for a whole year. After just a couple of weeks you'll begin to appreciate the benefits of a daily journal practice. Keeping a journal is highly regarded as one of the best things you can do to improve mindfulness and motivation. Take a look at the following examples of mocked up journal entry pages. This one depicts a typical day for me now. (See how the previous example progress chart corresponds with this journal entry on the relevant date of 12th of November.)

DATE Monday 12th November   **YEAR** 2018

FOOD: *What did you eat today?*

BREAKFAST: Porridge with almond milk & sunflower seeds

Snack: Banana, apple & satsuma, Vanilla protein shake

LUNCH: Baked beans on wholemeal toast

Snack: Avocado on rice cakes

DINNER: Homemade veggie burger, sweet potatoes & broccoli

Snack: Fresh Pineapple

DRINK: *What did you drink today?*

Any caffeinated drinks: Cappuccino with oat milk 1

Any alcoholic drinks: Small red wine 1

Any other drinks: Water ++++ Camomile tea 111 OJ 1

Any other drugs ingested: (including prescription, recreational, over the counter and nicotine) Paracetamol 11

QUICK CHECKLIST

WATER - how many litres? 3   MEDITATION - how many minutes? 3

SLEEP - how many hours? 8   EXERCISE - how many minutes? 60

LIFE EVENTS: *What happened today?*

Gym workout. Meeting with client. Dentist appointment.

Dinner with the family. Skype call with Steph in Australia.

Relaxed with a book in the bath. Early night.

EMOTIONS/THOUGHTS: *How did you feel today?*

Good, productive, calm, content.

Feeling happy & healthy in general.

Glad that I'm regularly practicing yoga again.

CONCERNS LIST: *What bothered you most today?*

Apprehensive about the next dentist appointment.

Hoping my client continues to be satisfied.

House move approaching - getting a bit stressed!

GRATITUDE LIST: *What are you most grateful for today?*

The next house is better, with a lovely garden.

Family are in good health.

Business is booming - so grateful!

And this mock up resembles a typical day for me from a few years ago. (It was around this time that I came up with the idea for this book, because necessity is the mother of invention.)

DATE *Monday 13th August* **YEAR** *2012*

FOOD: *What did you eat today?*

BREAKFAST: *Nothing*

Snack: *Chocolate*

LUNCH: *Fish & chips*

Snack: *Crisps*

DINNER: *Chinese takeaway*

Snack: *Cake*

DRINK: *What did you drink today?*

Any caffeinated drinks: *Tea IIII Coffee ↟↟↟ Coke I Red Bull I*

Any alcoholic drinks: *White wine IIII bottles of beer II G&T II*

Any other drinks: *Fanta I*

Any other drugs ingested: (including prescription, recreational, over the counter and nicotine) *Diazepam II*

Paracetamol III Cigarettes ↟↟↟ III

QUICK CHECKLIST

WATER how many litres? *1*   MEDITATION how many minutes? *0*

SLEEP - how many hours? *4*   EXERCISE - how many minutes? *0*

LIFE EVENTS: *What happened today?*

Woke up hungover from a heavy weekend

Work was crazy stressful - felt unproductive

Argued with boyfriend / went out for another work do

EMOTIONS/THOUGHTS: *How did you feel today?*

Felt exhausted, depressed, anxious & ill

Worried that I might lose my job

So tired of living this sort of unhealthy lifestyle

CONCERNS LIST: *What bothered you most today?*

Feel like I could lose my job if I carry on like this

Think my boyfriend wants to break up with me

Worried that I drink too much / feel unwell

GRATITUDE LIST: *What are you most grateful for today?*

Glad that I still have a job - just

Grateful that I haven't lost my relationship - yet

I still have hope that I can sort myself out

There are a few fundamental requirements that we all need to maintain in order to enjoy a baseline of general well-being. These fundamental necessities have nothing to do with personal preference or past experience. These basic needs apply to everyone: the need to continuously nourish ourselves with a well-balanced diet, the importance of daily exercise, the way we spend our time and how we interact with others, the importance of getting enough sleep and drinking enough water. These are all universal biological necessities and we disregard them at our peril. It stands to reason that if we fill our minds and bodies with rubbish, we'll end up feeling like rubbish. When we continuously starve ourselves of proper nourishment, physically, mentally and emotionally, we end up feeling drained, depressed and depleted. So many of us are worn to a frazzle, exhausted to the point of sickness, in desperate need of radical self-care and we don't even realise it. We are so used to feeling sick and tired that we've forgotten what it feels like to be healthy.

If you have any problem areas, (and I don't think there's a person on the planet who doesn't) you stand a better chance of being able to successfully address them if you've kept track of them and have an understanding of the things that influence them. It's only when we can truly see where a problem lies that we can take steps to do something about it. The Off The Rocks Journal is designed to help you do exactly that. If, after a few weeks of getting into the swing of routinely tracking your lifestyle choices, you want to take some steps to improve certain areas of your life, then you can, and you can monitor the results too.

Each day, after you've updated your progress chart, complete a fresh journal entry page. Simply fill out that day's information in the spaces provided. (See the examples previously provided.) The sections cover: what you ate, what you drank, your alcohol consumption, caffeine intake and any other drugs taken - including prescription, over the counter and nicotine. Basically, document everything you put into your body every day. This practice encourages and trains you to become more mindful, accountable and all-round health conscious. Coupled with the progress chart, over time you'll be able to easily identify any areas of your life that are 'on the rocks'. You'll also be in the perfect position to do something about it too should you want to.

Then there is also a quick checklist for:
• how many litres of water you drank that day
• how many hours of sleep you got that night
• how many minutes of meditation did you managed to fit in
• and how much exercise you did

There is space to briefly detail any life events that took place that day and another for you to record your emotions and thoughts for that day too. Finally, at the bottom of every page you are prompted to write down your top three current concerns for that day. (For example: a health worry, a work situation or a poorly pet). When you get your concerns off your chest and onto paper, you might find that you stop churning them over internally and instead start to look at them more objectively and constructively. This practice will encourage you to address the things that bother you in a more positive and practical way.

Last but not least, there is space to write the top three things that you feel most grateful for at that particular moment. (Perhaps: your gorgeous garden, a return to health after a bug or doing a job you love.) The benefits of writing a daily gratitude list have long been proven as one of the most rewarding things anyone can ever do for their mental health. It means cultivating an attitude of gratitude. Being in a steadier state of thankfulness rather than resentment. Learning to consistently look at things from a perspective of appreciation and abundance instead of dreary disappointment, longing and lack. As long as you're breathing there is always something to be grateful for. Even on your toughest days, if you look for things to be grateful for, you will find them. Over time, if you commit to it, this positive outlook will become your new normal - a happier, healthier normal. That's exactly what happened to me when I gave myself over to this process.

For best results, update your off the rocks journal and progress chart every day so that the information you record is crystal clear in your mind. The optimum times are either last thing at night for that day, or first thing in the morning - documenting information from the day before. It is absolutely imperative that you are completely honest with yourself. You will only see genuine results and progress if you record genuine information. We must all strive to take honest accountability for our own actions in life. We all get off track from time to time in one area or another, but you can decide to reclaim control of your life any time you like and The Off The Rocks Journal will help you to do so.

Where are you justifying your own bad behaviour? Where are you sabotaging yourself? What are you frightened of? You won't find the real answers to any of these universal questions unless you are truthful with yourself. It's time to drop the excuses that have held you back until now and accept that you can do things differently if you really want to. Your future will depend on the decisions you make today. You are capable of much more than you realise and the journey towards the life that you want is yours for the taking. You are always just one decision aways from a different outcome.

This book is not to be read once and chucked onto a shelf. This book is to be kept close. It's meant to be scribbled in, doodled on and lived through. Keep it handy on your bedside table or in your writing desk - anywhere you sit at some point each day. From this moment onwards, incorporate journaling into your existing daily routine. Break out your favourite ink pen. Try different coloured felt-tips to start plotting your charts. Add to this book every single day in your own lovely style of swirly handwriting. Make this book uniquely yours. Fill it to the brim with the glorious details of your everyday life and let it help you to understand yourself a little bit more.

Well, what are you waiting for, tiger? Let's get stuck in!

MONTH

ONE

<u>diet and exercise</u>

diet

It would be hard to overstate the importance of a healthy, well-balanced, nutritious diet. Every single food choice you ever make affects both your physical health and your mental heath. It impacts on how you function, how you feel and how you look. Everything we consume within our diet, both food and drink, healthy and unhealthy, will have an immediate effect and a longterm effect. Good nutrition is a vital part of a healthy lifestyle. Combined with exercise, a good diet will help you to attain and maintain a healthy weight, reduce your risk of chronic diseases and promote your overall physical and mental wellbeing. Good nutritional choices 90% of the time will result in good overall health. Poor nutritional choices 90% of the time will result in illness, lethargy, mood swings, poor sleep quality, depression, anxiety, countless diseases and premature death. Over 50% of the adult population in the UK alone are now considered overweight or obese and it's the number one reason that the NHS is under so much pressure. We have the knowledge and the power to help reverse this trend, but it starts with us and the very next decision we make with regards to what we choose to put into our bodies.

sugar

Around 1 in 4 adults in the UK are obese and it's costing the country a staggering £27 billion per year. In March 2016 for the first time ever the chancellor stepped in by introducing a sugar levy.

The most recent studies report that children consume three times the recommended amount of sugar on average and adults consume more than double.

The Scientific Advisory Committee on Nutrition (SACN) recently recommended that sugar should make up no more than 5% of daily calorie intake: 30g or 7 cubes of sugar maximum per day.

fat

Too much fat in your diet, especially saturated fats, raises cholesterol which increases the risk of heart disease. Experts agree that cutting down on all fats and replacing saturated fat with some unsaturated fat is the healthiest choice. Most people in the UK eat too much saturated fat. The population on average gets 12.6% of their energy (kJ/kcal) from saturated fats, which is slightly above the 11% maximum recommended by the government. The average man should aim to have no more than 30g of saturated fat per day and the average woman should aim to have no more than 20g of saturated fat per day. Children should consume less.

alcohol

The most recent UK government guidelines on safe* drinking limits recommend that both men and women do not exceed 14 units per week. This upper limit is meant to be spread out over the course of a week, ideally factoring in at least a couple of alcohol-free days.

One unit of alcohol is the equivalent to one of the following examples:
- A single measure of spirits (ABV 37.5%)
- A half a pint of average-strength (4%) lager
- A half a 175ml glass of average-strength (12%) wine

Or to put it in a more colloquial way, the weekly recommended upper limit would approximately translate to one of the following examples:
- 7 double gin and tonics - over the course of a week
- 7 pints of lager - over the course of a week
- Approximately one and a half bottles of wine - over the course of a week

Bear in mind that these are meant to be the *upper* weekly alcohol limits. You're not meant to *aim* for them. And you don't have to drink alcohol *at all* if you don't want to; more people than ever before are teetotal, sober curious or going sober for big chucks time each year. (There's a whole essay dedicated to alcohol further along in the book; given that the inclusion of it *and* the abstention from it is such an important part of so many people's lifestyles.)

*Health officials state that "there is no level of regular drinking that can be considered as completely safe".

exercise

As human beings, we are not meant to be sedentary all day long, and if we *are* for too much of the time, we begin to suffer for it. It really doesn't matter what sort of exercise you do as long as you do it. Do whatever you like and do it regularly. If it gets your body moving and your heart pumping, it's going to do you some good. Try to do something active and fairly intensive every day for *at least* 30 minutes. If you can do more, that's great. If you can improve on whatever you did yesterday, that's even better. There are thousands of ways to keep active so just find what suits you. You must be stronger than your excuses. You don't need a posh gym or a pushy trainer or the latest trendy class. You don't need any expensive equipment or special clothing. You don't want to be one of those people with all the gear and no idea, just get moving! Dancing around in your pants to your favourite songs in your bedroom is sometimes all we need to do. Just make sure you get out of breath and try to break a sweat. Do some push ups, lunges and jump squats. Make a note of what you did in The Off The Rocks Journal today and then improve on it tomorrow. Always strive to beat *your* personal best. Forget about how other people are doing, that's their business, not yours - to compare is to despair. Just keep your focus firmly on your own goals and your own gains and your own progress. You'll be smashing your PB's in no time.

The benefits of regular exercise are incredible: it increases energy levels, tones muscles, burns calories, aids digestion, improves brain function, enhances the immune system, promotes better sleep, improves mood, lowers anxiety, reduces depression, regulates hormones and helps to lower your risk from countless diseases. It's even better when you find a kind of exercise that you love, because then you can get fit *and* meet lots of lovely like-minded people whilst doing it too.

When it comes to exercise, absolutely anything is better than doing nothing. So get moving, get tracking and see how much better you look and feel after only a few weeks.

Future you will thank you for starting now.

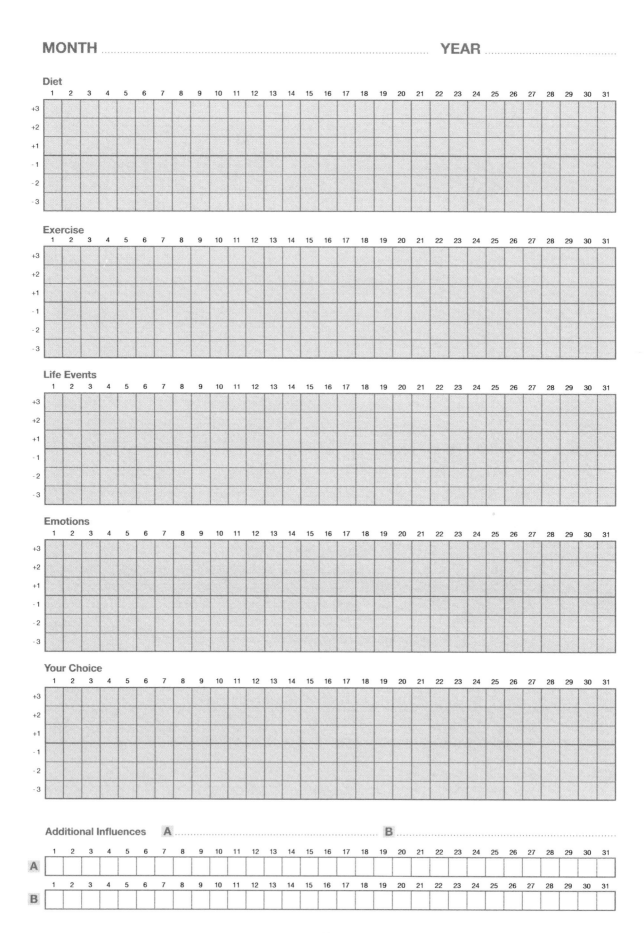

MONTH .... YEAR ....

Diet

Exercise

Life Events

Emotions

Your Choice

Additional Influences   A .... B ....

DATE .... **YEAR** ....

FOOD: *What did you eat today?*

BREAKFAST: ....

Snack: ....

LUNCH: ....

Snack: ....

DINNER: ....

Snack: ....

DRINK: *What did you drink today?*

Any caffeinated drinks: ....

Any alcoholic drinks: ....

Any other drinks: ....

Any other drugs ingested: (including prescription, recreational, over the counter and nicotine) ....

....

QUICK CHECKLIST

WATER - how many litres? ☐   MEDITATION - how many minutes? ☐

SLEEP - how many hours? ☐   EXERCISE - how many minutes? ☐

LIFE EVENTS: *What happened today?*

....

....

....

EMOTIONS/THOUGHTS: *How did you feel today?*

....

....

....

CONCERNS LIST: *What bothered you most today?*

....

....

....

GRATITUDE LIST: *What are you most grateful for today?*

....

....

....

DATE .... **YEAR** ....

FOOD: *What did you eat today?*

BREAKFAST: ....

Snack: ....

LUNCH: ....

Snack: ....

DINNER: ....

Snack: ....

DRINK: *What did you drink today?*

Any caffeinated drinks: ....

Any alcoholic drinks: ....

Any other drinks: ....

Any other drugs ingested: (including prescription, recreational, over the counter and nicotine) ....

....

QUICK CHECKLIST

WATER - how many litres? ▢   MEDITATION - how many minutes? ▢

SLEEP - how many hours? ▢   EXERCISE - how many minutes? ▢

LIFE EVENTS: *What happened today?*

....

....

....

EMOTIONS/THOUGHTS: *How did you feel today?*

....

....

....

CONCERNS LIST: *What bothered you most today?*

....

....

....

GRATITUDE LIST: *What are you most grateful for today?*

....

....

....

DATE .... **YEAR** ....

FOOD: *What did you eat today?*

BREAKFAST: ....

Snack: ....

LUNCH: ....

Snack: ....

DINNER: ....

Snack: ....

DRINK: *What did you drink today?*

Any caffeinated drinks: ....

Any alcoholic drinks: ....

Any other drinks: ....

Any other drugs ingested: (including prescription, recreational, over the counter and nicotine) ....

....

QUICK CHECKLIST

WATER - how many litres? ☐   MEDITATION - how many minutes? ☐

SLEEP - how many hours? ☐   EXERCISE - how many minutes? ☐

LIFE EVENTS: *What happened today?*

....

....

....

EMOTIONS/THOUGHTS: *How did you feel today?*

....

....

....

CONCERNS LIST: *What bothered you most today?*

....

....

....

GRATITUDE LIST: *What are you most grateful for today?*

....

....

....

DATE .... **YEAR** ....

FOOD: *What did you eat today?*

BREAKFAST: ....

Snack: ....

LUNCH: ....

Snack: ....

DINNER: ....

Snack: ....

DRINK: *What did you drink today?*

Any caffeinated drinks: ....

Any alcoholic drinks: ....

Any other drinks: ....

Any other drugs ingested: (including prescription, recreational, over the counter and nicotine) ....

....

QUICK CHECKLIST

WATER - how many litres?   ▢   MEDITATION - how many minutes?   ▢

SLEEP - how many hours?   ▢   EXERCISE - how many minutes?   ▢

LIFE EVENTS: *What happened today?*

....

....

....

EMOTIONS/THOUGHTS: *How did you feel today?*

....

....

....

CONCERNS LIST: *What bothered you most today?*

....

....

....

GRATITUDE LIST: *What are you most grateful for today?*

....

....

....

DATE .... **YEAR** ....

FOOD: *What did you eat today?*

BREAKFAST: ....

Snack: ....

LUNCH: ....

Snack: ....

DINNER: ....

Snack: ....

DRINK: *What did you drink today?*

Any caffeinated drinks: ....

Any alcoholic drinks: ....

Any other drinks: ....

Any other drugs ingested: (including prescription, recreational, over the counter and nicotine) ....

....

QUICK CHECKLIST

WATER - how many litres? ☐   MEDITATION - how many minutes? ☐

SLEEP - how many hours? ☐   EXERCISE - how many minutes? ☐

LIFE EVENTS: *What happened today?*

....

....

....

EMOTIONS/THOUGHTS: *How did you feel today?*

....

....

....

CONCERNS LIST: *What bothered you most today?*

....

....

....

GRATITUDE LIST: *What are you most grateful for today?*

....

....

....

DATE .... **YEAR** ....

FOOD: *What did you eat today?*

BREAKFAST: ....

Snack: ....

LUNCH: ....

Snack: ....

DINNER: ....

Snack: ....

DRINK: *What did you drink today?*

Any caffeinated drinks: ....

Any alcoholic drinks: ....

Any other drinks: ....

Any other drugs ingested: (including prescription, recreational, over the counter and nicotine) ....

....

QUICK CHECKLIST

WATER - how many litres? ▢   MEDITATION - how many minutes? ▢

SLEEP - how many hours? ▢   EXERCISE - how many minutes? ▢

LIFE EVENTS: *What happened today?*

....

....

....

EMOTIONS/THOUGHTS: *How did you feel today?*

....

....

....

CONCERNS LIST: *What bothered you most today?*

....

....

....

GRATITUDE LIST: *What are you most grateful for today?*

....

....

....

DATE .... **YEAR** ....

FOOD: *What did you eat today?*

BREAKFAST: ....

Snack: ....

LUNCH: ....

Snack: ....

DINNER: ....

Snack: ....

DRINK: *What did you drink today?*

Any caffeinated drinks: ....

Any alcoholic drinks: ....

Any other drinks: ....

Any other drugs ingested: (including prescription, recreational, over the counter and nicotine) ....

....

QUICK CHECKLIST

WATER - how many litres? ▨   MEDITATION - how many minutes? ▨

SLEEP - how many hours? ▨   EXERCISE - how many minutes? ▨

LIFE EVENTS: *What happened today?*

....

....

....

EMOTIONS/THOUGHTS: *How did you feel today?*

....

....

....

CONCERNS LIST: *What bothered you most today?*

....

....

....

GRATITUDE LIST: *What are you most grateful for today?*

....

....

....

DATE .... **YEAR** ....

FOOD: *What did you eat today?*

BREAKFAST: ....

Snack: ....

LUNCH: ....

Snack: ....

DINNER: ....

Snack: ....

DRINK: *What did you drink today?*

Any caffeinated drinks: ....

Any alcoholic drinks: ....

Any other drinks: ....

Any other drugs ingested: (including prescription, recreational, over the counter and nicotine) ....

....

QUICK CHECKLIST

WATER - how many litres? ☐   MEDITATION - how many minutes? ☐

SLEEP - how many hours? ☐   EXERCISE - how many minutes? ☐

LIFE EVENTS: *What happened today?*

....

....

....

EMOTIONS/THOUGHTS: *How did you feel today?*

....

....

....

CONCERNS LIST: *What bothered you most today?*

....

....

....

GRATITUDE LIST: *What are you most grateful for today?*

....

....

....

DATE .... **YEAR** ....

FOOD: *What did you eat today?*

BREAKFAST: ....

Snack: ....

LUNCH: ....

Snack: ....

DINNER: ....

Snack: ....

DRINK: *What did you drink today?*

Any caffeinated drinks: ....

Any alcoholic drinks: ....

Any other drinks: ....

Any other drugs ingested: (including prescription, recreational, over the counter and nicotine) ....

....

QUICK CHECKLIST

WATER - how many litres? ▨   MEDITATION - how many minutes? ▨

SLEEP - how many hours? ▨   EXERCISE - how many minutes? ▨

LIFE EVENTS: *What happened today?*

....

....

....

EMOTIONS/THOUGHTS: *How did you feel today?*

....

....

....

CONCERNS LIST: *What bothered you most today?*

....

....

....

GRATITUDE LIST: *What are you most grateful for today?*

....

....

....

DATE .... **YEAR** ....

FOOD: *What did you eat today?*

BREAKFAST: ....

Snack: ....

LUNCH: ....

Snack: ....

DINNER: ....

Snack: ....

DRINK: *What did you drink today?*

Any caffeinated drinks: ....

Any alcoholic drinks: ....

Any other drinks: ....

Any other drugs ingested: (including prescription, recreational, over the counter and nicotine) ....

....

QUICK CHECKLIST

WATER - how many litres? ☐   MEDITATION - how many minutes? ☐

SLEEP - how many hours? ☐   EXERCISE - how many minutes? ☐

LIFE EVENTS: *What happened today?*

....

....

....

EMOTIONS/THOUGHTS: *How did you feel today?*

....

....

....

CONCERNS LIST: *What bothered you most today?*

....

....

....

GRATITUDE LIST: *What are you most grateful for today?*

....

....

....

DATE .... **YEAR** ....

FOOD: *What did you eat today?*

BREAKFAST: ....

Snack: ....

LUNCH: ....

Snack: ....

DINNER: ....

Snack: ....

DRINK: *What did you drink today?*

Any caffeinated drinks: ....

Any alcoholic drinks: ....

Any other drinks: ....

Any other drugs ingested: (including prescription, recreational, over the counter and nicotine) ....

....

QUICK CHECKLIST

WATER - how many litres? ▨   MEDITATION - how many minutes? ▨

SLEEP - how many hours? ▨   EXERCISE - how many minutes? ▨

LIFE EVENTS: *What happened today?*

....

....

....

EMOTIONS/THOUGHTS: *How did you feel today?*

....

....

....

CONCERNS LIST: *What bothered you most today?*

....

....

....

GRATITUDE LIST: *What are you most grateful for today?*

....

....

....

DATE .... **YEAR** ....

FOOD: *What did you eat today?*

BREAKFAST: ....

Snack: ....

LUNCH: ....

Snack: ....

DINNER: ....

Snack: ....

DRINK: *What did you drink today?*

Any caffeinated drinks: ....

Any alcoholic drinks: ....

Any other drinks: ....

Any other drugs ingested: (including prescription, recreational, over the counter and nicotine) ....

....

QUICK CHECKLIST

WATER - how many litres?　　　　MEDITATION - how many minutes?

SLEEP - how many hours?　　　　EXERCISE - how many minutes?

LIFE EVENTS: *What happened today?*

....

....

....

EMOTIONS/THOUGHTS: *How did you feel today?*

....

....

....

CONCERNS LIST: *What bothered you most today?*

....

....

....

GRATITUDE LIST: *What are you most grateful for today?*

....

....

....

DATE .... **YEAR** ....

FOOD: *What did you eat today?*

BREAKFAST: ....

Snack: ....

LUNCH: ....

Snack: ....

DINNER: ....

Snack: ....

DRINK: *What did you drink today?*

Any caffeinated drinks: ....

Any alcoholic drinks: ....

Any other drinks: ....

Any other drugs ingested: (including prescription, recreational, over the counter and nicotine) ....

....

QUICK CHECKLIST

WATER - how many litres? ▢   MEDITATION - how many minutes? ▢

SLEEP - how many hours? ▢   EXERCISE - how many minutes? ▢

LIFE EVENTS: *What happened today?*

....

....

....

EMOTIONS/THOUGHTS: *How did you feel today?*

....

....

....

CONCERNS LIST: *What bothered you most today?*

....

....

....

GRATITUDE LIST: *What are you most grateful for today?*

....

....

....

DATE .... **YEAR** ....

FOOD: *What did you eat today?*

BREAKFAST: ....

Snack: ....

LUNCH: ....

Snack: ....

DINNER: ....

Snack: ....

DRINK: *What did you drink today?*

Any caffeinated drinks: ....

Any alcoholic drinks: ....

Any other drinks: ....

Any other drugs ingested: (including prescription, recreational, over the counter and nicotine) ....

....

QUICK CHECKLIST

WATER - how many litres? ☐   MEDITATION - how many minutes? ☐

SLEEP - how many hours? ☐   EXERCISE - how many minutes? ☐

LIFE EVENTS: *What happened today?*

....

....

....

EMOTIONS/THOUGHTS: *How did you feel today?*

....

....

....

CONCERNS LIST: *What bothered you most today?*

....

....

....

GRATITUDE LIST: *What are you most grateful for today?*

....

....

....

DATE .... **YEAR** ....

FOOD: *What did you eat today?*

BREAKFAST: ....

Snack: ....

LUNCH: ....

Snack: ....

DINNER: ....

Snack: ....

DRINK: *What did you drink today?*

Any caffeinated drinks: ....

Any alcoholic drinks: ....

Any other drinks: ....

Any other drugs ingested: (including prescription, recreational, over the counter and nicotine) ....

....

QUICK CHECKLIST

WATER - how many litres? ☐   MEDITATION - how many minutes? ☐

SLEEP - how many hours? ☐   EXERCISE - how many minutes? ☐

LIFE EVENTS: *What happened today?*

....

....

....

EMOTIONS/THOUGHTS: *How did you feel today?*

....

....

....

CONCERNS LIST: *What bothered you most today?*

....

....

....

GRATITUDE LIST: *What are you most grateful for today?*

....

....

....

DATE .... **YEAR** ....

FOOD: *What did you eat today?*

BREAKFAST: ....

Snack: ....

LUNCH: ....

Snack: ....

DINNER: ....

Snack: ....

DRINK: *What did you drink today?*

Any caffeinated drinks: ....

Any alcoholic drinks: ....

Any other drinks: ....

Any other drugs ingested: (including prescription, recreational, over the counter and nicotine) ....

....

QUICK CHECKLIST

WATER - how many litres?   MEDITATION - how many minutes?

SLEEP - how many hours?   EXERCISE - how many minutes?

LIFE EVENTS: *What happened today?*

....

....

....

EMOTIONS/THOUGHTS: *How did you feel today?*

....

....

....

CONCERNS LIST: *What bothered you most today?*

....

....

....

GRATITUDE LIST: *What are you most grateful for today?*

....

....

....

DATE .... **YEAR** ....

FOOD: *What did you eat today?*

BREAKFAST: ....

Snack: ....

LUNCH: ....

Snack: ....

DINNER: ....

Snack: ....

DRINK: *What did you drink today?*

Any caffeinated drinks: ....

Any alcoholic drinks: ....

Any other drinks: ....

Any other drugs ingested: (including prescription, recreational, over the counter and nicotine) ....

....

QUICK CHECKLIST

WATER - how many litres? ▢   MEDITATION - how many minutes? ▢

SLEEP - how many hours? ▢   EXERCISE - how many minutes? ▢

LIFE EVENTS: *What happened today?*

....

....

....

EMOTIONS/THOUGHTS: *How did you feel today?*

....

....

....

CONCERNS LIST: *What bothered you most today?*

....

....

....

GRATITUDE LIST: *What are you most grateful for today?*

....

....

....

DATE .... **YEAR** ....

FOOD: *What did you eat today?*

BREAKFAST: ....

Snack: ....

LUNCH: ....

Snack: ....

DINNER: ....

Snack: ....

DRINK: *What did you drink today?*

Any caffeinated drinks: ....

Any alcoholic drinks: ....

Any other drinks: ....

Any other drugs ingested: (including prescription, recreational, over the counter and nicotine) ....

....

QUICK CHECKLIST

WATER - how many litres? ☐   MEDITATION - how many minutes? ☐

SLEEP - how many hours? ☐   EXERCISE - how many minutes? ☐

LIFE EVENTS: *What happened today?*

....

....

....

EMOTIONS/THOUGHTS: *How did you feel today?*

....

....

....

CONCERNS LIST: *What bothered you most today?*

....

....

....

GRATITUDE LIST: *What are you most grateful for today?*

....

....

....

DATE .... **YEAR** ....

FOOD: *What did you eat today?*

BREAKFAST: ....

Snack: ....

LUNCH: ....

Snack: ....

DINNER: ....

Snack: ....

DRINK: *What did you drink today?*

Any caffeinated drinks: ....

Any alcoholic drinks: ....

Any other drinks: ....

Any other drugs ingested: (including prescription, recreational, over the counter and nicotine) ....

....

QUICK CHECKLIST

WATER - how many litres? ▢   MEDITATION - how many minutes? ▢

SLEEP - how many hours? ▢   EXERCISE - how many minutes? ▢

LIFE EVENTS: *What happened today?*

....

....

....

EMOTIONS/THOUGHTS: *How did you feel today?*

....

....

....

CONCERNS LIST: *What bothered you most today?*

....

....

....

GRATITUDE LIST: *What are you most grateful for today?*

....

....

....

DATE .... **YEAR** ....

FOOD: *What did you eat today?*

BREAKFAST: ....

Snack: ....

LUNCH: ....

Snack: ....

DINNER: ....

Snack: ....

DRINK: *What did you drink today?*

Any caffeinated drinks: ....

Any alcoholic drinks: ....

Any other drinks: ....

Any other drugs ingested: (including prescription, recreational, over the counter and nicotine) ....

....

QUICK CHECKLIST

WATER - how many litres? ☐   MEDITATION - how many minutes? ☐

SLEEP - how many hours? ☐   EXERCISE - how many minutes? ☐

LIFE EVENTS: *What happened today?*

....

....

....

EMOTIONS/THOUGHTS: *How did you feel today?*

....

....

....

CONCERNS LIST: *What bothered you most today?*

....

....

....

GRATITUDE LIST: *What are you most grateful for today?*

....

....

....

DATE .... **YEAR** ....

FOOD: *What did you eat today?*

BREAKFAST: ....

Snack: ....

LUNCH: ....

Snack: ....

DINNER: ....

Snack: ....

DRINK: *What did you drink today?*

Any caffeinated drinks: ....

Any alcoholic drinks: ....

Any other drinks: ....

Any other drugs ingested: (including prescription, recreational, over the counter and nicotine) ....

....

QUICK CHECKLIST

WATER - how many litres? ☐   MEDITATION - how many minutes? ☐

SLEEP - how many hours? ☐   EXERCISE - how many minutes? ☐

LIFE EVENTS: *What happened today?*

....

....

....

EMOTIONS/THOUGHTS: *How did you feel today?*

....

....

....

CONCERNS LIST: *What bothered you most today?*

....

....

....

GRATITUDE LIST: *What are you most grateful for today?*

....

....

....

DATE .... **YEAR** ....

FOOD: *What did you eat today?*

BREAKFAST: ....

Snack: ....

LUNCH: ....

Snack: ....

DINNER: ....

Snack: ....

DRINK: *What did you drink today?*

Any caffeinated drinks: ....

Any alcoholic drinks: ....

Any other drinks: ....

Any other drugs ingested: (including prescription, recreational, over the counter and nicotine) ....

....

QUICK CHECKLIST

WATER - how many litres? ☐   MEDITATION - how many minutes? ☐

SLEEP - how many hours? ☐   EXERCISE - how many minutes? ☐

LIFE EVENTS: *What happened today?*

....

....

....

EMOTIONS/THOUGHTS: *How did you feel today?*

....

....

....

CONCERNS LIST: *What bothered you most today?*

....

....

....

GRATITUDE LIST: *What are you most grateful for today?*

....

....

....

DATE .... **YEAR** ....

FOOD: *What did you eat today?*

BREAKFAST: ....

Snack: ....

LUNCH: ....

Snack: ....

DINNER: ....

Snack: ....

DRINK: *What did you drink today?*

Any caffeinated drinks: ....

Any alcoholic drinks: ....

Any other drinks: ....

Any other drugs ingested: (including prescription, recreational, over the counter and nicotine) ....

....

QUICK CHECKLIST

WATER - how many litres? ▨   MEDITATION - how many minutes? ▨

SLEEP - how many hours? ▨   EXERCISE - how many minutes? ▨

LIFE EVENTS: *What happened today?*

....

....

....

EMOTIONS/THOUGHTS: *How did you feel today?*

....

....

....

CONCERNS LIST: *What bothered you most today?*

....

....

....

GRATITUDE LIST: *What are you most grateful for today?*

....

....

....

DATE .... **YEAR** ....

FOOD: *What did you eat today?*

BREAKFAST: ....

Snack: ....

LUNCH: ....

Snack: ....

DINNER: ....

Snack: ....

DRINK: *What did you drink today?*

Any caffeinated drinks: ....

Any alcoholic drinks: ....

Any other drinks: ....

Any other drugs ingested: (including prescription, recreational, over the counter and nicotine) ....

....

QUICK CHECKLIST

WATER - how many litres? ▨   MEDITATION - how many minutes? ▨

SLEEP - how many hours? ▨   EXERCISE - how many minutes? ▨

LIFE EVENTS: *What happened today?*

....

....

....

EMOTIONS/THOUGHTS: *How did you feel today?*

....

....

....

CONCERNS LIST: *What bothered you most today?*

....

....

....

GRATITUDE LIST: *What are you most grateful for today?*

....

....

....

DATE .... **YEAR** ....

FOOD: *What did you eat today?*

BREAKFAST: ....

Snack: ....

LUNCH: ....

Snack: ....

DINNER: ....

Snack: ....

DRINK: *What did you drink today?*

Any caffeinated drinks: ....

Any alcoholic drinks: ....

Any other drinks: ....

Any other drugs ingested: (including prescription, recreational, over the counter and nicotine) ....

....

QUICK CHECKLIST

WATER - how many litres? ▧   MEDITATION - how many minutes? ▧

SLEEP - how many hours? ▧   EXERCISE - how many minutes? ▧

LIFE EVENTS: *What happened today?*

....

....

....

EMOTIONS/THOUGHTS: *How did you feel today?*

....

....

....

CONCERNS LIST: *What bothered you most today?*

....

....

....

GRATITUDE LIST: *What are you most grateful for today?*

....

....

....

DATE .... **YEAR** ....

FOOD: *What did you eat today?*

BREAKFAST: ....

Snack: ....

LUNCH: ....

Snack: ....

DINNER: ....

Snack: ....

DRINK: *What did you drink today?*

Any caffeinated drinks: ....

Any alcoholic drinks: ....

Any other drinks: ....

Any other drugs ingested: (including prescription, recreational, over the counter and nicotine) ....

....

QUICK CHECKLIST

WATER - how many litres? ▢   MEDITATION - how many minutes? ▢

SLEEP - how many hours? ▢   EXERCISE - how many minutes? ▢

LIFE EVENTS: *What happened today?*

....

....

....

EMOTIONS/THOUGHTS: *How did you feel today?*

....

....

....

CONCERNS LIST: *What bothered you most today?*

....

....

....

GRATITUDE LIST: *What are you most grateful for today?*

....

....

....

DATE .... **YEAR** ....

FOOD: *What did you eat today?*

BREAKFAST: ....

Snack: ....

LUNCH: ....

Snack: ....

DINNER: ....

Snack: ....

DRINK: *What did you drink today?*

Any caffeinated drinks: ....

Any alcoholic drinks: ....

Any other drinks: ....

Any other drugs ingested: (including prescription, recreational, over the counter and nicotine) ....

....

QUICK CHECKLIST

WATER - how many litres?　▢　　MEDITATION - how many minutes?　▢

SLEEP - how many hours?　▢　　EXERCISE - how many minutes?　▢

LIFE EVENTS: *What happened today?*

....

....

....

EMOTIONS/THOUGHTS: *How did you feel today?*

....

....

....

CONCERNS LIST: *What bothered you most today?*

....

....

....

GRATITUDE LIST: *What are you most grateful for today?*

....

....

....

DATE .... **YEAR** ....

FOOD: *What did you eat today?*

BREAKFAST: ....

Snack: ....

LUNCH: ....

Snack: ....

DINNER: ....

Snack: ....

DRINK: *What did you drink today?*

Any caffeinated drinks: ....

Any alcoholic drinks: ....

Any other drinks: ....

Any other drugs ingested: (including prescription, recreational, over the counter and nicotine) ....

....

QUICK CHECKLIST

WATER - how many litres? ▢   MEDITATION - how many minutes? ▢

SLEEP - how many hours? ▢   EXERCISE - how many minutes? ▢

LIFE EVENTS: *What happened today?*

....

....

....

EMOTIONS/THOUGHTS: *How did you feel today?*

....

....

....

CONCERNS LIST: *What bothered you most today?*

....

....

....

GRATITUDE LIST: *What are you most grateful for today?*

....

....

....

DATE .... **YEAR** ....

FOOD: *What did you eat today?*

BREAKFAST: ....

Snack: ....

LUNCH: ....

Snack: ....

DINNER: ....

Snack: ....

DRINK: *What did you drink today?*

Any caffeinated drinks: ....

Any alcoholic drinks: ....

Any other drinks: ....

Any other drugs ingested: (including prescription, recreational, over the counter and nicotine) ....

....

QUICK CHECKLIST

WATER - how many litres? ▢   MEDITATION - how many minutes? ▢

SLEEP - how many hours? ▢   EXERCISE - how many minutes? ▢

LIFE EVENTS: *What happened today?*

....

....

....

EMOTIONS/THOUGHTS: *How did you feel today?*

....

....

....

CONCERNS LIST: *What bothered you most today?*

....

....

....

GRATITUDE LIST: *What are you most grateful for today?*

....

....

....

DATE .... **YEAR** ....

FOOD: *What did you eat today?*

BREAKFAST: ....

Snack: ....

LUNCH: ....

Snack: ....

DINNER: ....

Snack: ....

DRINK: *What did you drink today?*

Any caffeinated drinks: ....

Any alcoholic drinks: ....

Any other drinks: ....

Any other drugs ingested: (including prescription, recreational, over the counter and nicotine) ....

....

QUICK CHECKLIST

WATER - how many litres? ▨   MEDITATION - how many minutes? ▨

SLEEP - how many hours? ▨   EXERCISE - how many minutes? ▨

LIFE EVENTS: *What happened today?*

....

....

....

EMOTIONS/THOUGHTS: *How did you feel today?*

....

....

....

CONCERNS LIST: *What bothered you most today?*

....

....

....

GRATITUDE LIST: *What are you most grateful for today?*

....

....

....

DATE .... YEAR ....

FOOD: *What did you eat today?*

BREAKFAST: ....

Snack: ....

LUNCH: ....

Snack: ....

DINNER: ....

Snack: ....

DRINK: *What did you drink today?*

Any caffeinated drinks: ....

Any alcoholic drinks: ....

Any other drinks: ....

Any other drugs ingested: (including prescription, recreational, over the counter and nicotine) ....

....

QUICK CHECKLIST

WATER - how many litres? ☐   MEDITATION - how many minutes? ☐

SLEEP - how many hours? ☐   EXERCISE - how many minutes? ☐

LIFE EVENTS: *What happened today?*

....

....

....

EMOTIONS/THOUGHTS: *How did you feel today?*

....

....

....

CONCERNS LIST: *What bothered you most today?*

....

....

....

GRATITUDE LIST: *What are you most grateful for today?*

....

....

....

MONTH TWO

<u>life events and emotions</u>

Significant life events are basically any disruptive occurrence or episode in your life. They can be positive or negative or a mixture of both. For instance, moving house can be pleasant and beneficial but it's often stressful too. Pulling muscles moving your furniture and filling out those pesky 'change of address' forms is no-one's idea of fun. Going on holiday is another mixed bag; guaranteed sunshine and a break from the usual routine is the pay off for mosquito bites and food poisoning. Getting married is lovely but it's also usually anxiety provoking. Having a baby is amazing but also understandably brings challenges, complications and concerns.

You get the idea - significant life events can be big or small, planned or unexpected, positive or negative. Problems at work, with your health, arguments with your partner; these are all life events worthy of being noted in The Off The Rocks Journal because they will have an effect on you, whether you are consciously aware of it or not. Whatever form they occur in, they still tend to cause your body to release stress chemicals such as adrenaline. Adrenaline can cause your autonomic nervous system to become more sensitive and this can affect the way your body reacts in all sorts of ways; a racing heart, high blood pressure, blood sugar crashes, mood swings and panic attacks.

Life is eventful and we all get anxious from time to time, none of us are immune from stress or the effect it has on us. The idea of this book is to help you to help yourself; to get to know yourself better. Understand your unique triggers. Learn to foresee your behavioural patterns. Save yourself from self-sabotage. Be more gentle with yourself in the ways that you need to be. And tougher with yourself in other ways. Get used to practicing radical self care and properly taking care of yourself. Be fully responsible for your own life. If you don't like something, change it. If you don't want to change it, stop making it someone else's problem. Become fully accountable for your own choices. If you don't want to do something, say no, politely and resolutely. If you want to do something, go and do it but only commit to doing it if you're going to accept the consequences. Create the life that you really want and truly get to know yourself along the way.

It's incredibly important to be aware of our emotions because these are the thoughts and feelings that we're conscious of and they are also often the driving force behind our motivations; both positive and negative.

Our emotions inform virtually all of our decision-making and life choices. They are also largely controllable, changeable and heavily influenced by the actions and thoughts that we allow ourselves to invest in. Our emotional state is a significant indicator of how healthy we are at any given time, both physically and mentally. Think back to the last time you felt highly emotional - perhaps cast your mind back to the last time you felt particularly angry or excited. Would you say that's you at your most reasonable and rational? No? Well, join the club.

If we regularly observe our emotions, and track them diligently and honestly, over time we'll begin to see our own individual patterns emerge. For instance, a lot of women find that at a certain point during their menstrual cycles (usually during the luteal phase) they'll become more emotionally attuned. A hyperawareness of not only their own feelings, but of other people's too. Their innate empathetic abilities level up - which is no bad thing. Conversely there are other points in the female cycle (often during the follicular phase) where a lot of women feel more energetic than usual; brimming with renewed strength and stamina. Pre-menopausal women also tend to crave protein, carbohydrate and iron sources at certain points for specific biological reasons too. Men also have their own hormonal profiles and biological imperatives that are distinct to their body chemistry too. The point is that when we understand ourselves more, we can take much better care of ourselves. If we can identify a pattern, we can predict it in advance, or at least recognise it when it occurs again. Once we're more familiar with something, we're also less afraid and more prepared. To be forewarned is to be forearmed.

When we take sure-footed steps in order to do things differently wherever needed, we become empowered and responsible, which will in turn contribute to a healthier, more robust and stable emotional state.

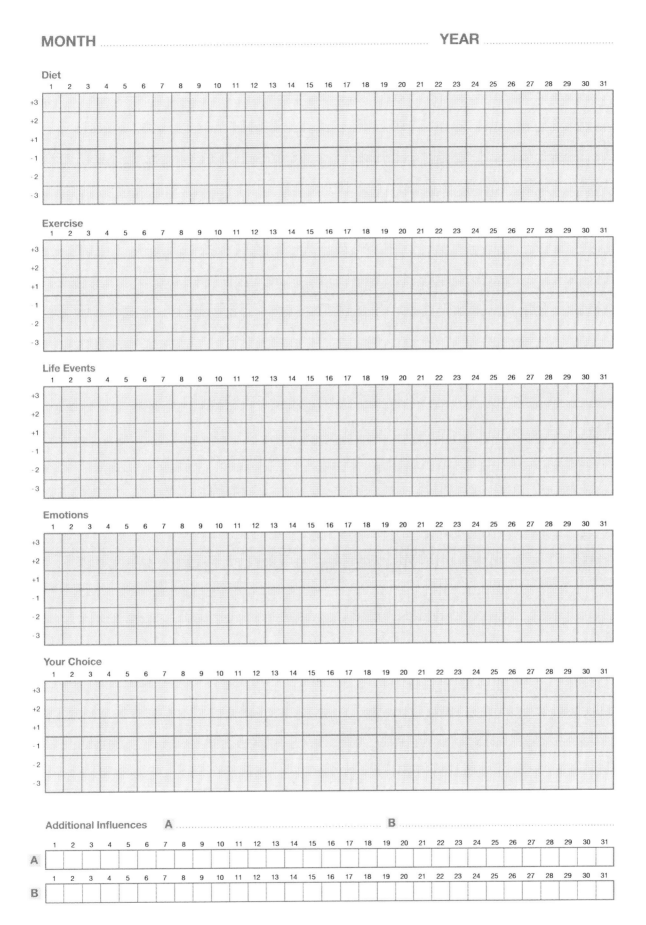

MONTH .... YEAR ....

Diet

Exercise

Life Events

Emotions

Your Choice

Additional Influences   A ....   B ....

A

B

DATE .... **YEAR** ....

FOOD: *What did you eat today?*

BREAKFAST: ....

Snack: ....

LUNCH: ....

Snack: ....

DINNER: ....

Snack: ....

DRINK: *What did you drink today?*

Any caffeinated drinks: ....

Any alcoholic drinks: ....

Any other drinks: ....

Any other drugs ingested: (including prescription, recreational, over the counter and nicotine) ....

....

QUICK CHECKLIST

WATER - how many litres? ▨   MEDITATION - how many minutes? ▨

SLEEP - how many hours? ▨   EXERCISE - how many minutes? ▨

LIFE EVENTS: *What happened today?*

....

....

....

EMOTIONS/THOUGHTS: *How did you feel today?*

....

....

....

CONCERNS LIST: *What bothered you most today?*

....

....

....

GRATITUDE LIST: *What are you most grateful for today?*

....

....

....

DATE .... **YEAR** ....

FOOD: *What did you eat today?*

BREAKFAST: ....

Snack: ....

LUNCH: ....

Snack: ....

DINNER: ....

Snack: ....

DRINK: *What did you drink today?*

Any caffeinated drinks: ....

Any alcoholic drinks: ....

Any other drinks: ....

Any other drugs ingested: (including prescription, recreational, over the counter and nicotine) ....

....

QUICK CHECKLIST

WATER - how many litres? ▨   MEDITATION - how many minutes? ▨

SLEEP - how many hours? ▨   EXERCISE - how many minutes? ▨

LIFE EVENTS: *What happened today?*

....

....

....

EMOTIONS/THOUGHTS: *How did you feel today?*

....

....

....

CONCERNS LIST: *What bothered you most today?*

....

....

....

GRATITUDE LIST: *What are you most grateful for today?*

....

....

....

FOOD: *What did you eat today?*

BREAKFAST: ....

Snack: ....

LUNCH: ....

Snack: ....

DINNER: ....

Snack: ....

DRINK: *What did you drink today?*

Any caffeinated drinks: ....

Any alcoholic drinks: ....

Any other drinks: ....

Any other drugs ingested: (including prescription, recreational, over the counter and nicotine) ....

....

QUICK CHECKLIST

WATER - how many litres? ☐   MEDITATION - how many minutes? ☐

SLEEP - how many hours? ☐   EXERCISE - how many minutes? ☐

LIFE EVENTS: *What happened today?*

....

....

....

EMOTIONS/THOUGHTS: *How did you feel today?*

....

....

....

CONCERNS LIST: *What bothered you most today?*

....

....

....

GRATITUDE LIST: *What are you most grateful for today?*

....

....

....

DATE .... **YEAR** ....

FOOD: *What did you eat today?*

BREAKFAST: ....

Snack: ....

LUNCH: ....

Snack: ....

DINNER: ....

Snack: ....

DRINK: *What did you drink today?*

Any caffeinated drinks: ....

Any alcoholic drinks: ....

Any other drinks: ....

Any other drugs ingested: (including prescription, recreational, over the counter and nicotine) ....

....

QUICK CHECKLIST

WATER - how many litres? ▢   MEDITATION - how many minutes? ▢

SLEEP - how many hours? ▢   EXERCISE - how many minutes? ▢

LIFE EVENTS: *What happened today?*

....

....

....

EMOTIONS/THOUGHTS: *How did you feel today?*

....

....

....

CONCERNS LIST: *What bothered you most today?*

....

....

....

GRATITUDE LIST: *What are you most grateful for today?*

....

....

....

DATE .... **YEAR** ....

FOOD: *What did you eat today?*

BREAKFAST: ....

Snack: ....

LUNCH: ....

Snack: ....

DINNER: ....

Snack: ....

DRINK: *What did you drink today?*

Any caffeinated drinks: ....

Any alcoholic drinks: ....

Any other drinks: ....

Any other drugs ingested: (including prescription, recreational, over the counter and nicotine) ....

....

QUICK CHECKLIST

WATER - how many litres? ☐   MEDITATION - how many minutes? ☐

SLEEP - how many hours? ☐   EXERCISE - how many minutes? ☐

LIFE EVENTS: *What happened today?*

....

....

....

EMOTIONS/THOUGHTS: *How did you feel today?*

....

....

....

CONCERNS LIST: *What bothered you most today?*

....

....

....

GRATITUDE LIST: *What are you most grateful for today?*

....

....

....

DATE .... **YEAR** ....

FOOD: *What did you eat today?*

BREAKFAST: ....

Snack: ....

LUNCH: ....

Snack: ....

DINNER: ....

Snack: ....

DRINK: *What did you drink today?*

Any caffeinated drinks: ....

Any alcoholic drinks: ....

Any other drinks: ....

Any other drugs ingested: (including prescription, recreational, over the counter and nicotine) ....

....

QUICK CHECKLIST

WATER - how many litres? ▢   MEDITATION - how many minutes? ▢

SLEEP - how many hours? ▢   EXERCISE - how many minutes? ▢

LIFE EVENTS: *What happened today?*

....

....

....

EMOTIONS/THOUGHTS: *How did you feel today?*

....

....

....

CONCERNS LIST: *What bothered you most today?*

....

....

....

GRATITUDE LIST: *What are you most grateful for today?*

....

....

....

DATE .... YEAR ....

FOOD: *What did you eat today?*

BREAKFAST: ....

Snack: ....

LUNCH: ....

Snack: ....

DINNER: ....

Snack: ....

DRINK: *What did you drink today?*

Any caffeinated drinks: ....

Any alcoholic drinks: ....

Any other drinks: ....

Any other drugs ingested: (including prescription, recreational, over the counter and nicotine) ....

....

QUICK CHECKLIST

WATER - how many litres? ☐   MEDITATION - how many minutes? ☐

SLEEP - how many hours? ☐   EXERCISE - how many minutes? ☐

LIFE EVENTS: *What happened today?*

....

....

....

EMOTIONS/THOUGHTS: *How did you feel today?*

....

....

....

CONCERNS LIST: *What bothered you most today?*

....

....

....

GRATITUDE LIST: *What are you most grateful for today?*

....

....

....

DATE .... **YEAR** ....

FOOD: *What did you eat today?*

BREAKFAST: ....

Snack: ....

LUNCH: ....

Snack: ....

DINNER: ....

Snack: ....

DRINK: *What did you drink today?*

Any caffeinated drinks: ....

Any alcoholic drinks: ....

Any other drinks: ....

Any other drugs ingested: (including prescription, recreational, over the counter and nicotine) ....

....

QUICK CHECKLIST

WATER - how many litres? ☐   MEDITATION - how many minutes? ☐

SLEEP - how many hours? ☐   EXERCISE - how many minutes? ☐

LIFE EVENTS: *What happened today?*

....

....

....

EMOTIONS/THOUGHTS: *How did you feel today?*

....

....

....

CONCERNS LIST: *What bothered you most today?*

....

....

....

GRATITUDE LIST: *What are you most grateful for today?*

....

....

....

DATE .... **YEAR** ....

FOOD: *What did you eat today?*

BREAKFAST: ....

Snack: ....

LUNCH: ....

Snack: ....

DINNER: ....

Snack: ....

DRINK: *What did you drink today?*

Any caffeinated drinks: ....

Any alcoholic drinks: ....

Any other drinks: ....

Any other drugs ingested: (including prescription, recreational, over the counter and nicotine) ....

....

QUICK CHECKLIST

WATER - how many litres? ☐   MEDITATION - how many minutes? ☐

SLEEP - how many hours? ☐   EXERCISE - how many minutes? ☐

LIFE EVENTS: *What happened today?*

....

....

....

EMOTIONS/THOUGHTS: *How did you feel today?*

....

....

....

CONCERNS LIST: *What bothered you most today?*

....

....

....

GRATITUDE LIST: *What are you most grateful for today?*

....

....

....

DATE .... **YEAR** ....

FOOD: *What did you eat today?*

BREAKFAST: ....

Snack: ....

LUNCH: ....

Snack: ....

DINNER: ....

Snack: ....

DRINK: *What did you drink today?*

Any caffeinated drinks: ....

Any alcoholic drinks: ....

Any other drinks: ....

Any other drugs ingested: (including prescription, recreational, over the counter and nicotine) ....

....

QUICK CHECKLIST

WATER - how many litres? ☐   MEDITATION - how many minutes? ☐

SLEEP - how many hours? ☐   EXERCISE - how many minutes? ☐

LIFE EVENTS: *What happened today?*

....

....

....

EMOTIONS/THOUGHTS: *How did you feel today?*

....

....

....

CONCERNS LIST: *What bothered you most today?*

....

....

....

GRATITUDE LIST: *What are you most grateful for today?*

....

....

....

DATE .... **YEAR** ....

FOOD: *What did you eat today?*

BREAKFAST: ....

Snack: ....

LUNCH: ....

Snack: ....

DINNER: ....

Snack: ....

DRINK: *What did you drink today?*

Any caffeinated drinks: ....

Any alcoholic drinks: ....

Any other drinks: ....

Any other drugs ingested: (including prescription, recreational, over the counter and nicotine) ....

....

QUICK CHECKLIST

WATER - how many litres? [ ]   MEDITATION - how many minutes? [ ]

SLEEP - how many hours? [ ]   EXERCISE - how many minutes? [ ]

LIFE EVENTS: *What happened today?*

....

....

....

EMOTIONS/THOUGHTS: *How did you feel today?*

....

....

....

CONCERNS LIST: *What bothered you most today?*

....

....

....

GRATITUDE LIST: *What are you most grateful for today?*

....

....

....

DATE .... **YEAR** ....

FOOD: *What did you eat today?*

BREAKFAST: ....

Snack: ....

LUNCH: ....

Snack: ....

DINNER: ....

Snack: ....

DRINK: *What did you drink today?*

Any caffeinated drinks: ....

Any alcoholic drinks: ....

Any other drinks: ....

Any other drugs ingested: (including prescription, recreational, over the counter and nicotine) ....

....

QUICK CHECKLIST

WATER - how many litres? ☐   MEDITATION - how many minutes? ☐

SLEEP - how many hours? ☐   EXERCISE - how many minutes? ☐

LIFE EVENTS: *What happened today?*

....

....

....

EMOTIONS/THOUGHTS: *How did you feel today?*

....

....

....

CONCERNS LIST: *What bothered you most today?*

....

....

....

GRATITUDE LIST: *What are you most grateful for today?*

....

....

....

DATE .... **YEAR** ....

FOOD: *What did you eat today?*

BREAKFAST: ....

Snack: ....

LUNCH: ....

Snack: ....

DINNER: ....

Snack: ....

DRINK: *What did you drink today?*

Any caffeinated drinks: ....

Any alcoholic drinks: ....

Any other drinks: ....

Any other drugs ingested: (including prescription, recreational, over the counter and nicotine) ....

....

QUICK CHECKLIST

WATER - how many litres? ⬜   MEDITATION - how many minutes? ⬜

SLEEP - how many hours? ⬜   EXERCISE - how many minutes? ⬜

LIFE EVENTS: *What happened today?*

....

....

....

EMOTIONS/THOUGHTS: *How did you feel today?*

....

....

....

CONCERNS LIST: *What bothered you most today?*

....

....

....

GRATITUDE LIST: *What are you most grateful for today?*

....

....

....

DATE .... **YEAR** ....

FOOD: *What did you eat today?*

BREAKFAST: ....

Snack: ....

LUNCH: ....

Snack: ....

DINNER: ....

Snack: ....

DRINK: *What did you drink today?*

Any caffeinated drinks: ....

Any alcoholic drinks: ....

Any other drinks: ....

Any other drugs ingested: (including prescription, recreational, over the counter and nicotine) ....

....

QUICK CHECKLIST

WATER - how many litres? ☐   MEDITATION - how many minutes? ☐

SLEEP - how many hours? ☐   EXERCISE - how many minutes? ☐

LIFE EVENTS: *What happened today?*

....

....

....

EMOTIONS/THOUGHTS: *How did you feel today?*

....

....

....

CONCERNS LIST: *What bothered you most today?*

....

....

....

GRATITUDE LIST: *What are you most grateful for today?*

....

....

....

DATE .... **YEAR** ....

FOOD: *What did you eat today?*

BREAKFAST: ....

Snack: ....

LUNCH: ....

Snack: ....

DINNER: ....

Snack: ....

DRINK: *What did you drink today?*

Any caffeinated drinks: ....

Any alcoholic drinks: ....

Any other drinks: ....

Any other drugs ingested: (including prescription, recreational, over the counter and nicotine) ....

....

QUICK CHECKLIST

WATER - how many litres?   ▨   MEDITATION - how many minutes?   ▨

SLEEP - how many hours?   ▨   EXERCISE - how many minutes?   ▨

LIFE EVENTS: *What happened today?*

....

....

....

EMOTIONS/THOUGHTS: *How did you feel today?*

....

....

....

CONCERNS LIST: *What bothered you most today?*

....

....

....

GRATITUDE LIST: *What are you most grateful for today?*

....

....

....

DATE .... **YEAR** ....

FOOD: *What did you eat today?*

BREAKFAST: ....

Snack: ....

LUNCH: ....

Snack: ....

DINNER: ....

Snack: ....

DRINK: *What did you drink today?*

Any caffeinated drinks: ....

Any alcoholic drinks: ....

Any other drinks: ....

Any other drugs ingested: (including prescription, recreational, over the counter and nicotine) ....

....

QUICK CHECKLIST

WATER - how many litres? ▨   MEDITATION - how many minutes? ▨

SLEEP - how many hours? ▨   EXERCISE - how many minutes? ▨

LIFE EVENTS: *What happened today?*

....

....

....

EMOTIONS/THOUGHTS: *How did you feel today?*

....

....

....

CONCERNS LIST: *What bothered you most today?*

....

....

....

GRATITUDE LIST: *What are you most grateful for today?*

....

....

....

DATE .... **YEAR** ....

FOOD: *What did you eat today?*

BREAKFAST: ....

Snack: ....

LUNCH: ....

Snack: ....

DINNER: ....

Snack: ....

DRINK: *What did you drink today?*

Any caffeinated drinks: ....

Any alcoholic drinks: ....

Any other drinks: ....

Any other drugs ingested: (including prescription, recreational, over the counter and nicotine) ....

....

QUICK CHECKLIST

WATER - how many litres? ▢   MEDITATION - how many minutes? ▢

SLEEP - how many hours? ▢   EXERCISE - how many minutes? ▢

LIFE EVENTS: *What happened today?*

....

....

....

EMOTIONS/THOUGHTS: *How did you feel today?*

....

....

....

CONCERNS LIST: *What bothered you most today?*

....

....

....

GRATITUDE LIST: *What are you most grateful for today?*

....

....

....

DATE .... **YEAR** ....

FOOD: *What did you eat today?*

BREAKFAST: ....

Snack: ....

LUNCH: ....

Snack: ....

DINNER: ....

Snack: ....

DRINK: *What did you drink today?*

Any caffeinated drinks: ....

Any alcoholic drinks: ....

Any other drinks: ....

Any other drugs ingested: (including prescription, recreational, over the counter and nicotine) ....

....

QUICK CHECKLIST

WATER - how many litres? ☐   MEDITATION - how many minutes? ☐

SLEEP - how many hours? ☐   EXERCISE - how many minutes? ☐

LIFE EVENTS: *What happened today?*

....

....

....

EMOTIONS/THOUGHTS: *How did you feel today?*

....

....

....

CONCERNS LIST: *What bothered you most today?*

....

....

....

GRATITUDE LIST: *What are you most grateful for today?*

....

....

....

DATE .... **YEAR** ....

FOOD: *What did you eat today?*

BREAKFAST: ....

Snack: ....

LUNCH: ....

Snack: ....

DINNER: ....

Snack: ....

DRINK: *What did you drink today?*

Any caffeinated drinks: ....

Any alcoholic drinks: ....

Any other drinks: ....

Any other drugs ingested: (including prescription, recreational, over the counter and nicotine) ....

....

QUICK CHECKLIST

WATER - how many litres? ☐   MEDITATION - how many minutes? ☐

SLEEP - how many hours? ☐   EXERCISE - how many minutes? ☐

LIFE EVENTS: *What happened today?*

....

....

....

EMOTIONS/THOUGHTS: *How did you feel today?*

....

....

....

CONCERNS LIST: *What bothered you most today?*

....

....

....

GRATITUDE LIST: *What are you most grateful for today?*

....

....

....

DATE .... **YEAR** ....

FOOD: *What did you eat today?*

BREAKFAST: ....

Snack: ....

LUNCH: ....

Snack: ....

DINNER: ....

Snack: ....

DRINK: *What did you drink today?*

Any caffeinated drinks: ....

Any alcoholic drinks: ....

Any other drinks: ....

Any other drugs ingested: (including prescription, recreational, over the counter and nicotine) ....

....

QUICK CHECKLIST

WATER - how many litres?　▦　　MEDITATION - how many minutes?　▦

SLEEP - how many hours?　▦　　EXERCISE - how many minutes?　▦

LIFE EVENTS: *What happened today?*

....

....

....

EMOTIONS/THOUGHTS: *How did you feel today?*

....

....

....

CONCERNS LIST: *What bothered you most today?*

....

....

....

GRATITUDE LIST: *What are you most grateful for today?*

....

....

....

DATE .... **YEAR** ....

FOOD: *What did you eat today?*

BREAKFAST: ....

Snack: ....

LUNCH: ....

Snack: ....

DINNER: ....

Snack: ....

DRINK: *What did you drink today?*

Any caffeinated drinks: ....

Any alcoholic drinks: ....

Any other drinks: ....

Any other drugs ingested: (including prescription, recreational, over the counter and nicotine) ....

....

QUICK CHECKLIST

WATER - how many litres? ☐   MEDITATION - how many minutes? ☐

SLEEP - how many hours? ☐   EXERCISE - how many minutes? ☐

LIFE EVENTS: *What happened today?*

....

....

....

EMOTIONS/THOUGHTS: *How did you feel today?*

....

....

....

CONCERNS LIST: *What bothered you most today?*

....

....

....

GRATITUDE LIST: *What are you most grateful for today?*

....

....

....

DATE .... **YEAR** ....

FOOD: *What did you eat today?*

BREAKFAST: ....

Snack: ....

LUNCH: ....

Snack: ....

DINNER: ....

Snack: ....

DRINK: *What did you drink today?*

Any caffeinated drinks: ....

Any alcoholic drinks: ....

Any other drinks: ....

Any other drugs ingested: (including prescription, recreational, over the counter and nicotine) ....

....

QUICK CHECKLIST

WATER - how many litres? ☐   MEDITATION - how many minutes? ☐

SLEEP - how many hours? ☐   EXERCISE - how many minutes? ☐

LIFE EVENTS: *What happened today?*

....

....

....

EMOTIONS/THOUGHTS: *How did you feel today?*

....

....

....

CONCERNS LIST: *What bothered you most today?*

....

....

....

GRATITUDE LIST: *What are you most grateful for today?*

....

....

....

DATE .... **YEAR** ....

FOOD: *What did you eat today?*

BREAKFAST: ....

Snack: ....

LUNCH: ....

Snack: ....

DINNER: ....

Snack: ....

DRINK: *What did you drink today?*

Any caffeinated drinks: ....

Any alcoholic drinks: ....

Any other drinks: ....

Any other drugs ingested: (including prescription, recreational, over the counter and nicotine) ....

....

QUICK CHECKLIST

WATER - how many litres? ☐   MEDITATION - how many minutes? ☐

SLEEP - how many hours? ☐   EXERCISE - how many minutes? ☐

LIFE EVENTS: *What happened today?*

....

....

....

EMOTIONS/THOUGHTS: *How did you feel today?*

....

....

....

CONCERNS LIST: *What bothered you most today?*

....

....

....

GRATITUDE LIST: *What are you most grateful for today?*

....

....

....

DATE .... **YEAR** ....

FOOD: *What did you eat today?*

BREAKFAST: ....

Snack: ....

LUNCH: ....

Snack: ....

DINNER: ....

Snack: ....

DRINK: *What did you drink today?*

Any caffeinated drinks: ....

Any alcoholic drinks: ....

Any other drinks: ....

Any other drugs ingested: (including prescription, recreational, over the counter and nicotine) ....

....

QUICK CHECKLIST

WATER - how many litres? ☐   MEDITATION - how many minutes? ☐

SLEEP - how many hours? ☐   EXERCISE - how many minutes? ☐

LIFE EVENTS: *What happened today?*

....

....

....

EMOTIONS/THOUGHTS: *How did you feel today?*

....

....

....

CONCERNS LIST: *What bothered you most today?*

....

....

....

GRATITUDE LIST: *What are you most grateful for today?*

....

....

....

DATE .... **YEAR** ....

FOOD: *What did you eat today?*

BREAKFAST: ....

Snack: ....

LUNCH: ....

Snack: ....

DINNER: ....

Snack: ....

DRINK: *What did you drink today?*

Any caffeinated drinks: ....

Any alcoholic drinks: ....

Any other drinks: ....

Any other drugs ingested: (including prescription, recreational, over the counter and nicotine) ....

....

QUICK CHECKLIST

WATER - how many litres? ▢   MEDITATION - how many minutes? ▢

SLEEP - how many hours? ▢   EXERCISE - how many minutes? ▢

LIFE EVENTS: *What happened today?*

....

....

....

EMOTIONS/THOUGHTS: *How did you feel today?*

....

....

....

CONCERNS LIST: *What bothered you most today?*

....

....

....

GRATITUDE LIST: *What are you most grateful for today?*

....

....

....

DATE .... **YEAR** ....

FOOD: *What did you eat today?*

BREAKFAST: ....

Snack: ....

LUNCH: ....

Snack: ....

DINNER: ....

Snack: ....

DRINK: *What did you drink today?*

Any caffeinated drinks: ....

Any alcoholic drinks: ....

Any other drinks: ....

Any other drugs ingested: (including prescription, recreational, over the counter and nicotine) ....

....

QUICK CHECKLIST

WATER - how many litres? ▨   MEDITATION - how many minutes? ▨

SLEEP - how many hours? ▨   EXERCISE - how many minutes? ▨

LIFE EVENTS: *What happened today?*

....

....

....

EMOTIONS/THOUGHTS: *How did you feel today?*

....

....

....

CONCERNS LIST: *What bothered you most today?*

....

....

....

GRATITUDE LIST: *What are you most grateful for today?*

....

....

....

DATE .... **YEAR** ....

FOOD: *What did you eat today?*

BREAKFAST: ....

Snack: ....

LUNCH: ....

Snack: ....

DINNER: ....

Snack: ....

DRINK: *What did you drink today?*

Any caffeinated drinks: ....

Any alcoholic drinks: ....

Any other drinks: ....

Any other drugs ingested: (including prescription, recreational, over the counter and nicotine) ....

....

QUICK CHECKLIST

WATER - how many litres? ☐   MEDITATION - how many minutes? ☐

SLEEP - how many hours? ☐   EXERCISE - how many minutes? ☐

LIFE EVENTS: *What happened today?*

....

....

....

EMOTIONS/THOUGHTS: *How did you feel today?*

....

....

....

CONCERNS LIST: *What bothered you most today?*

....

....

....

GRATITUDE LIST: *What are you most grateful for today?*

....

....

....

DATE .... **YEAR** ....

FOOD: *What did you eat today?*

BREAKFAST: ....

Snack: ....

LUNCH: ....

Snack: ....

DINNER: ....

Snack: ....

DRINK: *What did you drink today?*

Any caffeinated drinks: ....

Any alcoholic drinks: ....

Any other drinks: ....

Any other drugs ingested: (including prescription, recreational, over the counter and nicotine) ....

....

QUICK CHECKLIST

WATER - how many litres? ☐   MEDITATION - how many minutes? ☐

SLEEP - how many hours? ☐   EXERCISE - how many minutes? ☐

LIFE EVENTS: *What happened today?*

....

....

....

EMOTIONS/THOUGHTS: *How did you feel today?*

....

....

....

CONCERNS LIST: *What bothered you most today?*

....

....

....

GRATITUDE LIST: *What are you most grateful for today?*

....

....

....

DATE .... **YEAR** ....

FOOD: *What did you eat today?*

BREAKFAST: ....

Snack: ....

LUNCH: ....

Snack: ....

DINNER: ....

Snack: ....

DRINK: *What did you drink today?*

Any caffeinated drinks: ....

Any alcoholic drinks: ....

Any other drinks: ....

Any other drugs ingested: (including prescription, recreational, over the counter and nicotine) ....

....

QUICK CHECKLIST

WATER - how many litres? ☐   MEDITATION - how many minutes? ☐

SLEEP - how many hours? ☐   EXERCISE - how many minutes? ☐

LIFE EVENTS: *What happened today?*

....

....

....

EMOTIONS/THOUGHTS: *How did you feel today?*

....

....

....

CONCERNS LIST: *What bothered you most today?*

....

....

....

GRATITUDE LIST: *What are you most grateful for today?*

....

....

....

DATE .... **YEAR** ....

FOOD: *What did you eat today?*

BREAKFAST: ....

Snack: ....

LUNCH: ....

Snack: ....

DINNER: ....

Snack: ....

DRINK: *What did you drink today?*

Any caffeinated drinks: ....

Any alcoholic drinks: ....

Any other drinks: ....

Any other drugs ingested: (including prescription, recreational, over the counter and nicotine) ....

....

QUICK CHECKLIST

WATER - how many litres? ☐   MEDITATION - how many minutes? ☐

SLEEP - how many hours? ☐   EXERCISE - how many minutes? ☐

LIFE EVENTS: *What happened today?*

....

....

....

EMOTIONS/THOUGHTS: *How did you feel today?*

....

....

....

CONCERNS LIST: *What bothered you most today?*

....

....

....

GRATITUDE LIST: *What are you most grateful for today?*

....

....

....

DATE .... **YEAR** ....

FOOD: *What did you eat today?*

BREAKFAST: ....

Snack: ....

LUNCH: ....

Snack: ....

DINNER: ....

Snack: ....

DRINK: *What did you drink today?*

Any caffeinated drinks: ....

Any alcoholic drinks: ....

Any other drinks: ....

Any other drugs ingested: (including prescription, recreational, over the counter and nicotine) ....

....

QUICK CHECKLIST

WATER - how many litres? ⬜   MEDITATION - how many minutes? ⬜

SLEEP - how many hours? ⬜   EXERCISE - how many minutes? ⬜

LIFE EVENTS: *What happened today?*

....

....

....

EMOTIONS/THOUGHTS: *How did you feel today?*

....

....

....

CONCERNS LIST: *What bothered you most today?*

....

....

....

GRATITUDE LIST: *What are you most grateful for today?*

....

....

....

MONTH THREE

<u>acting out</u>

Whenever you act out, meaning: whenever you find yourself acting outside of a healthy boundary; binge-drinking, chain-smoking over-eating or developing co-dependent relationships for example, it's incredibly helpful to understand those behaviours if you're serious about changing them. To identify the patterns, triggers and the underlying reasons that drive you towards them in the first place. The Off The Rocks Journal is a fantastic tool for helping you to uncover your own patterns, triggers and drivers.

When problem behaviour goes on unabated, it often gets progressively worse over time rather than better. This is how a bad habit becomes a dependency and at some point, that habitual over-reliance can be aptly described as an addiction. When this sort of destructive behaviour isn't fully understood or addressed, it's often justified, ignored and repeated indefinitely until something catastrophic occurs. Perhaps you'll put yourself in danger, or have an accident or a near miss, maybe you'll put someone else at risk, make yourself ill, lose a job or damage your most valued relationships. There's no end to the ways in which we can cause disruption, damage and destruction to ourselves and others when we're not taking proper care of ourselves.

People often reach a point where they feel sufficiently dreadful enough to make some changes. This is where the proverbial concept of 'rock bottom' comes from, but you don't have to wait until a problem gets even worse before you address your problem areas. You can change the trajectory of your life any time you want. Listen, mush, there is no amount of suffering you have to endure before you can make the decision to turn things around.

You can walk away of your own accord *before* you're forced to run.

We can get so entrenched in our behavioural pattens that change feels impossible, but feelings are not facts. And habits, even long-standing, deep-rooted ones, can be replaced with healthy alternatives. There is no 'one way' of doing this, but there are endless possibilities and there is infinite hope.

MONTH .... YEAR ....

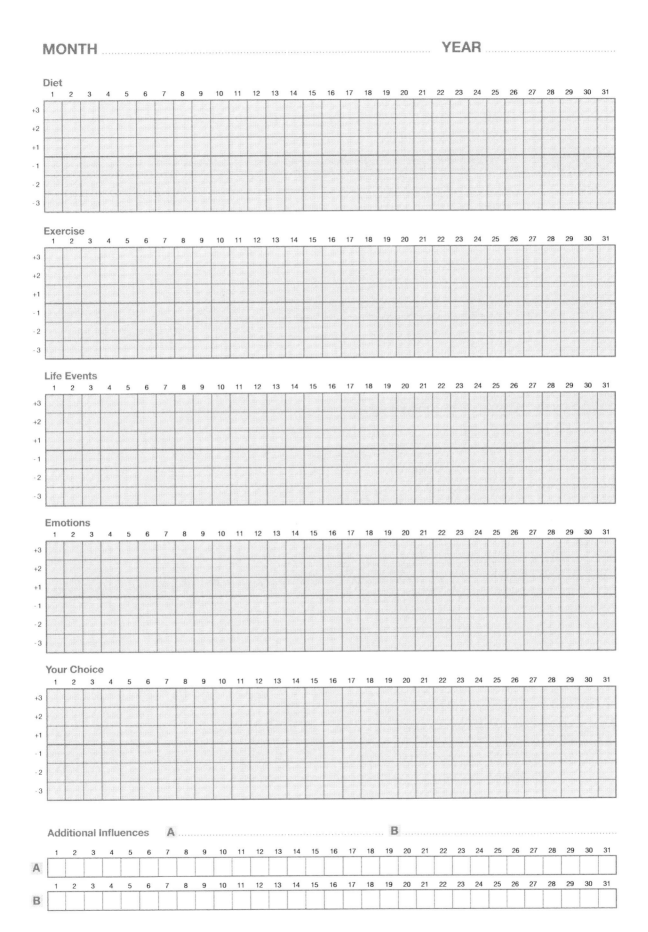

Diet

Exercise

Life Events

Emotions

Your Choice

Additional Influences   A ....   B ....

DATE .... YEAR ....

FOOD: *What did you eat today?*

BREAKFAST: ....

Snack: ....

LUNCH: ....

Snack: ....

DINNER: ....

Snack: ....

DRINK: *What did you drink today?*

Any caffeinated drinks: ....

Any alcoholic drinks: ....

Any other drinks: ....

Any other drugs ingested: (including prescription, recreational, over the counter and nicotine) ....

....

QUICK CHECKLIST

WATER - how many litres? ☐   MEDITATION - how many minutes? ☐

SLEEP - how many hours? ☐   EXERCISE - how many minutes? ☐

LIFE EVENTS: *What happened today?*

....

....

....

EMOTIONS/THOUGHTS: *How did you feel today?*

....

....

....

CONCERNS LIST: *What bothered you most today?*

....

....

....

GRATITUDE LIST: *What are you most grateful for today?*

....

....

....

DATE .... **YEAR** ....

FOOD: *What did you eat today?*

BREAKFAST: ....

Snack: ....

LUNCH: ....

Snack: ....

DINNER: ....

Snack: ....

DRINK: *What did you drink today?*

Any caffeinated drinks: ....

Any alcoholic drinks: ....

Any other drinks: ....

Any other drugs ingested: (including prescription, recreational, over the counter and nicotine) ....

....

QUICK CHECKLIST

WATER - how many litres? ☐   MEDITATION - how many minutes? ☐

SLEEP - how many hours? ☐   EXERCISE - how many minutes? ☐

LIFE EVENTS: *What happened today?*

....

....

....

EMOTIONS/THOUGHTS: *How did you feel today?*

....

....

....

CONCERNS LIST: *What bothered you most today?*

....

....

....

GRATITUDE LIST: *What are you most grateful for today?*

....

....

....

DATE .... YEAR ....

FOOD: *What did you eat today?*

BREAKFAST: ....

Snack: ....

LUNCH: ....

Snack: ....

DINNER: ....

Snack: ....

DRINK: *What did you drink today?*

Any caffeinated drinks: ....

Any alcoholic drinks: ....

Any other drinks: ....

Any other drugs ingested: (including prescription, recreational, over the counter and nicotine) ....

....

QUICK CHECKLIST

WATER - how many litres? ☐   MEDITATION - how many minutes? ☐

SLEEP - how many hours? ☐   EXERCISE - how many minutes? ☐

LIFE EVENTS: *What happened today?*

....

....

....

EMOTIONS/THOUGHTS: *How did you feel today?*

....

....

....

CONCERNS LIST: *What bothered you most today?*

....

....

....

GRATITUDE LIST: *What are you most grateful for today?*

....

....

....

DATE .... **YEAR** ....

FOOD: *What did you eat today?*

BREAKFAST: ....

Snack: ....

LUNCH: ....

Snack: ....

DINNER: ....

Snack: ....

DRINK: *What did you drink today?*

Any caffeinated drinks: ....

Any alcoholic drinks: ....

Any other drinks: ....

Any other drugs ingested: (including prescription, recreational, over the counter and nicotine) ....

....

QUICK CHECKLIST

WATER - how many litres? ▢   MEDITATION - how many minutes? ▢

SLEEP - how many hours? ▢   EXERCISE - how many minutes? ▢

LIFE EVENTS: *What happened today?*

....

....

....

EMOTIONS/THOUGHTS: *How did you feel today?*

....

....

....

CONCERNS LIST: *What bothered you most today?*

....

....

....

GRATITUDE LIST: *What are you most grateful for today?*

....

....

....

DATE .... **YEAR** ....

FOOD: *What did you eat today?*

BREAKFAST: ....

Snack: ....

LUNCH: ....

Snack: ....

DINNER: ....

Snack: ....

DRINK: *What did you drink today?*

Any caffeinated drinks: ....

Any alcoholic drinks: ....

Any other drinks: ....

Any other drugs ingested: (including prescription, recreational, over the counter and nicotine) ....

....

QUICK CHECKLIST

WATER - how many litres? ☐   MEDITATION - how many minutes? ☐

SLEEP - how many hours? ☐   EXERCISE - how many minutes? ☐

LIFE EVENTS: *What happened today?*

....

....

....

EMOTIONS/THOUGHTS: *How did you feel today?*

....

....

....

CONCERNS LIST: *What bothered you most today?*

....

....

....

GRATITUDE LIST: *What are you most grateful for today?*

....

....

....

DATE .... **YEAR** ....

FOOD: *What did you eat today?*

BREAKFAST: ....

Snack: ....

LUNCH: ....

Snack: ....

DINNER: ....

Snack: ....

DRINK: *What did you drink today?*

Any caffeinated drinks: ....

Any alcoholic drinks: ....

Any other drinks: ....

Any other drugs ingested: (including prescription, recreational, over the counter and nicotine) ....

....

QUICK CHECKLIST

WATER - how many litres? ☐   MEDITATION - how many minutes? ☐

SLEEP - how many hours? ☐   EXERCISE - how many minutes? ☐

LIFE EVENTS: *What happened today?*

....

....

....

EMOTIONS/THOUGHTS: *How did you feel today?*

....

....

....

CONCERNS LIST: *What bothered you most today?*

....

....

....

GRATITUDE LIST: *What are you most grateful for today?*

....

....

....

DATE .... **YEAR** ....

FOOD: *What did you eat today?*

BREAKFAST: ....

Snack: ....

LUNCH: ....

Snack: ....

DINNER: ....

Snack: ....

DRINK: *What did you drink today?*

Any caffeinated drinks: ....

Any alcoholic drinks: ....

Any other drinks: ....

Any other drugs ingested: (including prescription, recreational, over the counter and nicotine) ....

....

QUICK CHECKLIST

WATER - how many litres? ☐   MEDITATION - how many minutes? ☐

SLEEP - how many hours? ☐   EXERCISE - how many minutes? ☐

LIFE EVENTS: *What happened today?*

....

....

....

EMOTIONS/THOUGHTS: *How did you feel today?*

....

....

....

CONCERNS LIST: *What bothered you most today?*

....

....

....

GRATITUDE LIST: *What are you most grateful for today?*

....

....

....

DATE .... **YEAR** ....

FOOD: *What did you eat today?*

BREAKFAST: ....

Snack: ....

LUNCH: ....

Snack: ....

DINNER: ....

Snack: ....

DRINK: *What did you drink today?*

Any caffeinated drinks: ....

Any alcoholic drinks: ....

Any other drinks: ....

Any other drugs ingested: (including prescription, recreational, over the counter and nicotine) ....

....

QUICK CHECKLIST

WATER - how many litres? ▦   MEDITATION - how many minutes? ▦

SLEEP - how many hours? ▦   EXERCISE - how many minutes? ▦

LIFE EVENTS: *What happened today?*

....

....

....

EMOTIONS/THOUGHTS: *How did you feel today?*

....

....

....

CONCERNS LIST: *What bothered you most today?*

....

....

....

GRATITUDE LIST: *What are you most grateful for today?*

....

....

....

DATE .... **YEAR** ....

FOOD: *What did you eat today?*

BREAKFAST: ....

Snack: ....

LUNCH: ....

Snack: ....

DINNER: ....

Snack: ....

DRINK: *What did you drink today?*

Any caffeinated drinks: ....

Any alcoholic drinks: ....

Any other drinks: ....

Any other drugs ingested: (including prescription, recreational, over the counter and nicotine) ....

....

QUICK CHECKLIST

WATER - how many litres? ☐   MEDITATION - how many minutes? ☐

SLEEP - how many hours? ☐   EXERCISE - how many minutes? ☐

LIFE EVENTS: *What happened today?*

....

....

....

EMOTIONS/THOUGHTS: *How did you feel today?*

....

....

....

CONCERNS LIST: *What bothered you most today?*

....

....

....

GRATITUDE LIST: *What are you most grateful for today?*

....

....

....

DATE .... **YEAR** ....

FOOD: *What did you eat today?*

BREAKFAST: ....

Snack: ....

LUNCH: ....

Snack: ....

DINNER: ....

Snack: ....

DRINK: *What did you drink today?*

Any caffeinated drinks: ....

Any alcoholic drinks: ....

Any other drinks: ....

Any other drugs ingested: (including prescription, recreational, over the counter and nicotine) ....

....

QUICK CHECKLIST

WATER - how many litres?　▨　　MEDITATION - how many minutes?　▨

SLEEP - how many hours?　▨　　EXERCISE - how many minutes?　▨

LIFE EVENTS: *What happened today?*

....

....

....

EMOTIONS/THOUGHTS: *How did you feel today?*

....

....

....

CONCERNS LIST: *What bothered you most today?*

....

....

....

GRATITUDE LIST: *What are you most grateful for today?*

....

....

....

DATE .... **YEAR** ....

FOOD: *What did you eat today?*

BREAKFAST: ....

Snack: ....

LUNCH: ....

Snack: ....

DINNER: ....

Snack: ....

DRINK: *What did you drink today?*

Any caffeinated drinks: ....

Any alcoholic drinks: ....

Any other drinks: ....

Any other drugs ingested: (including prescription, recreational, over the counter and nicotine) ....

....

QUICK CHECKLIST

WATER - how many litres? ☐   MEDITATION - how many minutes? ☐

SLEEP - how many hours? ☐   EXERCISE - how many minutes? ☐

LIFE EVENTS: *What happened today?*

....

....

....

EMOTIONS/THOUGHTS: *How did you feel today?*

....

....

....

CONCERNS LIST: *What bothered you most today?*

....

....

....

GRATITUDE LIST: *What are you most grateful for today?*

....

....

....

DATE .... **YEAR** ....

FOOD: *What did you eat today?*

BREAKFAST: ....

Snack: ....

LUNCH: ....

Snack: ....

DINNER: ....

Snack: ....

DRINK: *What did you drink today?*

Any caffeinated drinks: ....

Any alcoholic drinks: ....

Any other drinks: ....

Any other drugs ingested: (including prescription, recreational, over the counter and nicotine) ....

....

QUICK CHECKLIST

WATER - how many litres? ▨   MEDITATION - how many minutes? ▨

SLEEP - how many hours? ▨   EXERCISE - how many minutes? ▨

LIFE EVENTS: *What happened today?*

....

....

....

EMOTIONS/THOUGHTS: *How did you feel today?*

....

....

....

CONCERNS LIST: *What bothered you most today?*

....

....

....

GRATITUDE LIST: *What are you most grateful for today?*

....

....

....

DATE .... **YEAR** ....

FOOD: *What did you eat today?*

BREAKFAST: ....

Snack: ....

LUNCH: ....

Snack: ....

DINNER: ....

Snack: ....

DRINK: *What did you drink today?*

Any caffeinated drinks: ....

Any alcoholic drinks: ....

Any other drinks: ....

Any other drugs ingested: (including prescription, recreational, over the counter and nicotine) ....

....

QUICK CHECKLIST

WATER - how many litres? ☐   MEDITATION - how many minutes? ☐

SLEEP - how many hours? ☐   EXERCISE - how many minutes? ☐

LIFE EVENTS: *What happened today?*

....

....

....

EMOTIONS/THOUGHTS: *How did you feel today?*

....

....

....

CONCERNS LIST: *What bothered you most today?*

....

....

....

GRATITUDE LIST: *What are you most grateful for today?*

....

....

....

DATE .... **YEAR** ....

FOOD: *What did you eat today?*

BREAKFAST: ....

Snack: ....

LUNCH: ....

Snack: ....

DINNER: ....

Snack: ....

DRINK: *What did you drink today?*

Any caffeinated drinks: ....

Any alcoholic drinks: ....

Any other drinks: ....

Any other drugs ingested: (including prescription, recreational, over the counter and nicotine) ....

....

QUICK CHECKLIST

WATER - how many litres? ▓   MEDITATION - how many minutes? ▓

SLEEP - how many hours? ▓   EXERCISE - how many minutes? ▓

LIFE EVENTS: *What happened today?*

....

....

....

EMOTIONS/THOUGHTS: *How did you feel today?*

....

....

....

CONCERNS LIST: *What bothered you most today?*

....

....

....

GRATITUDE LIST: *What are you most grateful for today?*

....

....

....

DATE .... YEAR ....

FOOD: *What did you eat today?*

BREAKFAST: ....

Snack: ....

LUNCH: ....

Snack: ....

DINNER: ....

Snack: ....

DRINK: *What did you drink today?*

Any caffeinated drinks: ....

Any alcoholic drinks: ....

Any other drinks: ....

Any other drugs ingested: (including prescription, recreational, over the counter and nicotine) ....

....

QUICK CHECKLIST

WATER - how many litres? ▢   MEDITATION - how many minutes? ▢

SLEEP - how many hours? ▢   EXERCISE - how many minutes? ▢

LIFE EVENTS: *What happened today?*

....

....

....

EMOTIONS/THOUGHTS: *How did you feel today?*

....

....

....

CONCERNS LIST: *What bothered you most today?*

....

....

....

GRATITUDE LIST: *What are you most grateful for today?*

....

....

....

DATE .... **YEAR** ....

FOOD: *What did you eat today?*

BREAKFAST: ....

Snack: ....

LUNCH: ....

Snack: ....

DINNER: ....

Snack: ....

DRINK: *What did you drink today?*

Any caffeinated drinks: ....

Any alcoholic drinks: ....

Any other drinks: ....

Any other drugs ingested: (including prescription, recreational, over the counter and nicotine) ....

....

QUICK CHECKLIST

WATER - how many litres? ▥   MEDITATION - how many minutes? ▥

SLEEP - how many hours? ▥   EXERCISE - how many minutes? ▥

LIFE EVENTS: *What happened today?*

....

....

....

EMOTIONS/THOUGHTS: *How did you feel today?*

....

....

....

CONCERNS LIST: *What bothered you most today?*

....

....

....

GRATITUDE LIST: *What are you most grateful for today?*

....

....

....

DATE .... **YEAR** ....

FOOD: *What did you eat today?*

BREAKFAST: ....

Snack: ....

LUNCH: ....

Snack: ....

DINNER: ....

Snack: ....

DRINK: *What did you drink today?*

Any caffeinated drinks: ....

Any alcoholic drinks: ....

Any other drinks: ....

Any other drugs ingested: (including prescription, recreational, over the counter and nicotine) ....

....

QUICK CHECKLIST

WATER - how many litres?   ▦   MEDITATION - how many minutes?   ▦

SLEEP - how many hours?   ▦   EXERCISE - how many minutes?   ▦

LIFE EVENTS: *What happened today?*

....

....

....

EMOTIONS/THOUGHTS: *How did you feel today?*

....

....

....

CONCERNS LIST: *What bothered you most today?*

....

....

....

GRATITUDE LIST: *What are you most grateful for today?*

....

....

....

DATE .... **YEAR** ....

FOOD: *What did you eat today?*

BREAKFAST: ....

Snack: ....

LUNCH: ....

Snack: ....

DINNER: ....

Snack: ....

DRINK: *What did you drink today?*

Any caffeinated drinks: ....

Any alcoholic drinks: ....

Any other drinks: ....

Any other drugs ingested: (including prescription, recreational, over the counter and nicotine) ....

....

QUICK CHECKLIST

WATER - how many litres? ☐   MEDITATION - how many minutes? ☐

SLEEP - how many hours? ☐   EXERCISE - how many minutes? ☐

LIFE EVENTS: *What happened today?*

....

....

....

EMOTIONS/THOUGHTS: *How did you feel today?*

....

....

....

CONCERNS LIST: *What bothered you most today?*

....

....

....

GRATITUDE LIST: *What are you most grateful for today?*

....

....

....

DATE .... **YEAR** ....

FOOD: *What did you eat today?*

BREAKFAST: ....

Snack: ....

LUNCH: ....

Snack: ....

DINNER: ....

Snack: ....

DRINK: *What did you drink today?*

Any caffeinated drinks: ....

Any alcoholic drinks: ....

Any other drinks: ....

Any other drugs ingested: (including prescription, recreational, over the counter and nicotine) ....

....

QUICK CHECKLIST

WATER - how many litres? ▨   MEDITATION - how many minutes? ▨

SLEEP - how many hours? ▨   EXERCISE - how many minutes? ▨

LIFE EVENTS: *What happened today?*

....

....

....

EMOTIONS/THOUGHTS: *How did you feel today?*

....

....

....

CONCERNS LIST: *What bothered you most today?*

....

....

....

GRATITUDE LIST: *What are you most grateful for today?*

....

....

....

DATE .... **YEAR** ....

FOOD: *What did you eat today?*

BREAKFAST: ....

Snack: ....

LUNCH: ....

Snack: ....

DINNER: ....

Snack: ....

DRINK: *What did you drink today?*

Any caffeinated drinks: ....

Any alcoholic drinks: ....

Any other drinks: ....

Any other drugs ingested: (including prescription, recreational, over the counter and nicotine) ....

....

QUICK CHECKLIST

WATER - how many litres? ▨   MEDITATION - how many minutes? ▨

SLEEP - how many hours? ▨   EXERCISE - how many minutes? ▨

LIFE EVENTS: *What happened today?*

....

....

....

EMOTIONS/THOUGHTS: *How did you feel today?*

....

....

....

CONCERNS LIST: *What bothered you most today?*

....

....

....

GRATITUDE LIST: *What are you most grateful for today?*

....

....

....

DATE .... **YEAR** ....

FOOD: *What did you eat today?*

BREAKFAST: ....

Snack: ....

LUNCH: ....

Snack: ....

DINNER: ....

Snack: ....

DRINK: *What did you drink today?*

Any caffeinated drinks: ....

Any alcoholic drinks: ....

Any other drinks: ....

Any other drugs ingested: (including prescription, recreational, over the counter and nicotine) ....

....

QUICK CHECKLIST

WATER - how many litres? ☐   MEDITATION - how many minutes? ☐

SLEEP - how many hours? ☐   EXERCISE - how many minutes? ☐

LIFE EVENTS: *What happened today?*

....

....

....

EMOTIONS/THOUGHTS: *How did you feel today?*

....

....

....

CONCERNS LIST: *What bothered you most today?*

....

....

....

GRATITUDE LIST: *What are you most grateful for today?*

....

....

....

DATE .... **YEAR** ....

FOOD: *What did you eat today?*

BREAKFAST: ....

Snack: ....

LUNCH: ....

Snack: ....

DINNER: ....

Snack: ....

DRINK: *What did you drink today?*

Any caffeinated drinks: ....

Any alcoholic drinks: ....

Any other drinks: ....

Any other drugs ingested: (including prescription, recreational, over the counter and nicotine) ....
....

QUICK CHECKLIST

WATER - how many litres? ▓   MEDITATION - how many minutes? ▓

SLEEP - how many hours? ▓   EXERCISE - how many minutes? ▓

LIFE EVENTS: *What happened today?*

....
....
....

EMOTIONS/THOUGHTS: *How did you feel today?*

....
....
....

CONCERNS LIST: *What bothered you most today?*

....
....
....

GRATITUDE LIST: *What are you most grateful for today?*

....
....
....

DATE .... **YEAR** ....

FOOD: *What did you eat today?*

BREAKFAST: ....

Snack: ....

LUNCH: ....

Snack: ....

DINNER: ....

Snack: ....

DRINK: *What did you drink today?*

Any caffeinated drinks: ....

Any alcoholic drinks: ....

Any other drinks: ....

Any other drugs ingested: (including prescription, recreational, over the counter and nicotine) ....

....

QUICK CHECKLIST

WATER - how many litres? ☐   MEDITATION - how many minutes? ☐

SLEEP - how many hours? ☐   EXERCISE - how many minutes? ☐

LIFE EVENTS: *What happened today?*

....

....

....

EMOTIONS/THOUGHTS: *How did you feel today?*

....

....

....

CONCERNS LIST: *What bothered you most today?*

....

....

....

GRATITUDE LIST: *What are you most grateful for today?*

....

....

....

DATE .... **YEAR** ....

FOOD: *What did you eat today?*

BREAKFAST: ....

Snack: ....

LUNCH: ....

Snack: ....

DINNER: ....

Snack: ....

DRINK: *What did you drink today?*

Any caffeinated drinks: ....

Any alcoholic drinks: ....

Any other drinks: ....

Any other drugs ingested: (including prescription, recreational, over the counter and nicotine) ....

....

QUICK CHECKLIST

WATER - how many litres? ☐ MEDITATION - how many minutes? ☐

SLEEP - how many hours? ☐ EXERCISE - how many minutes? ☐

LIFE EVENTS: *What happened today?*

....

....

....

EMOTIONS/THOUGHTS: *How did you feel today?*

....

....

....

CONCERNS LIST: *What bothered you most today?*

....

....

....

GRATITUDE LIST: *What are you most grateful for today?*

....

....

....

DATE .... **YEAR** ....

FOOD: *What did you eat today?*

BREAKFAST: ....

Snack: ....

LUNCH: ....

Snack: ....

DINNER: ....

Snack: ....

DRINK: *What did you drink today?*

Any caffeinated drinks: ....

Any alcoholic drinks: ....

Any other drinks: ....

Any other drugs ingested: (including prescription, recreational, over the counter and nicotine) ....

....

QUICK CHECKLIST

WATER - how many litres?　▦　　MEDITATION - how many minutes?　▦

SLEEP - how many hours?　▦　　EXERCISE - how many minutes?　▦

LIFE EVENTS: *What happened today?*

....

....

....

EMOTIONS/THOUGHTS: *How did you feel today?*

....

....

....

CONCERNS LIST: *What bothered you most today?*

....

....

....

GRATITUDE LIST: *What are you most grateful for today?*

....

....

....

DATE .... **YEAR** ....

FOOD: *What did you eat today?*

BREAKFAST: ....

Snack: ....

LUNCH: ....

Snack: ....

DINNER: ....

Snack: ....

DRINK: *What did you drink today?*

Any caffeinated drinks: ....

Any alcoholic drinks: ....

Any other drinks: ....

Any other drugs ingested: (including prescription, recreational, over the counter and nicotine) ....

....

QUICK CHECKLIST

WATER - how many litres? ▢   MEDITATION - how many minutes? ▢

SLEEP - how many hours? ▢   EXERCISE - how many minutes? ▢

LIFE EVENTS: *What happened today?*

....

....

....

EMOTIONS/THOUGHTS: *How did you feel today?*

....

....

....

CONCERNS LIST: *What bothered you most today?*

....

....

....

GRATITUDE LIST: *What are you most grateful for today?*

....

....

....

DATE .... **YEAR** ....

FOOD: *What did you eat today?*

BREAKFAST: ....

Snack: ....

LUNCH: ....

Snack: ....

DINNER: ....

Snack: ....

DRINK: *What did you drink today?*

Any caffeinated drinks: ....

Any alcoholic drinks: ....

Any other drinks: ....

Any other drugs ingested: (including prescription, recreational, over the counter and nicotine) ....

....

QUICK CHECKLIST

WATER - how many litres?   ☐   MEDITATION - how many minutes?   ☐

SLEEP - how many hours?   ☐   EXERCISE - how many minutes?   ☐

LIFE EVENTS: *What happened today?*

....

....

....

EMOTIONS/THOUGHTS: *How did you feel today?*

....

....

....

CONCERNS LIST: *What bothered you most today?*

....

....

....

GRATITUDE LIST: *What are you most grateful for today?*

....

....

....

DATE .... **YEAR** ....

FOOD: *What did you eat today?*

BREAKFAST: ....

Snack: ....

LUNCH: ....

Snack: ....

DINNER: ....

Snack: ....

DRINK: *What did you drink today?*

Any caffeinated drinks: ....

Any alcoholic drinks: ....

Any other drinks: ....

Any other drugs ingested: (including prescription, recreational, over the counter and nicotine) ....

....

QUICK CHECKLIST

WATER - how many litres? ☐   MEDITATION - how many minutes? ☐

SLEEP - how many hours? ☐   EXERCISE - how many minutes? ☐

LIFE EVENTS: *What happened today?*

....

....

....

EMOTIONS/THOUGHTS: *How did you feel today?*

....

....

....

CONCERNS LIST: *What bothered you most today?*

....

....

....

GRATITUDE LIST: *What are you most grateful for today?*

....

....

....

DATE .... YEAR ....

FOOD: *What did you eat today?*

BREAKFAST: ....

Snack: ....

LUNCH: ....

Snack: ....

DINNER: ....

Snack: ....

DRINK: *What did you drink today?*

Any caffeinated drinks: ....

Any alcoholic drinks: ....

Any other drinks: ....

Any other drugs ingested: (including prescription, recreational, over the counter and nicotine) ....

....

QUICK CHECKLIST

WATER - how many litres? ☐   MEDITATION - how many minutes? ☐

SLEEP - how many hours? ☐   EXERCISE - how many minutes? ☐

LIFE EVENTS: *What happened today?*

....

....

....

EMOTIONS/THOUGHTS: *How did you feel today?*

....

....

....

CONCERNS LIST: *What bothered you most today?*

....

....

....

GRATITUDE LIST: *What are you most grateful for today?*

....

....

....

DATE .... **YEAR** ....

FOOD: *What did you eat today?*

BREAKFAST: ....

Snack: ....

LUNCH: ....

Snack: ....

DINNER: ....

Snack: ....

DRINK: *What did you drink today?*

Any caffeinated drinks: ....

Any alcoholic drinks: ....

Any other drinks: ....

Any other drugs ingested: (including prescription, recreational, over the counter and nicotine) ....

....

QUICK CHECKLIST

WATER - how many litres? ▨   MEDITATION - how many minutes? ▨

SLEEP - how many hours? ▨   EXERCISE - how many minutes? ▨

LIFE EVENTS: *What happened today?*

....

....

....

EMOTIONS/THOUGHTS: *How did you feel today?*

....

....

....

CONCERNS LIST: *What bothered you most today?*

....

....

....

GRATITUDE LIST: *What are you most grateful for today?*

....

....

....

DATE .... **YEAR** ....

FOOD: *What did you eat today?*

BREAKFAST: ....

Snack: ....

LUNCH: ....

Snack: ....

DINNER: ....

Snack: ....

DRINK: *What did you drink today?*

Any caffeinated drinks: ....

Any alcoholic drinks: ....

Any other drinks: ....

Any other drugs ingested: (including prescription, recreational, over the counter and nicotine) ....

....

QUICK CHECKLIST

WATER - how many litres? ▢   MEDITATION - how many minutes? ▢

SLEEP - how many hours? ▢   EXERCISE - how many minutes? ▢

LIFE EVENTS: *What happened today?*

....

....

....

EMOTIONS/THOUGHTS: *How did you feel today?*

....

....

....

CONCERNS LIST: *What bothered you most today?*

....

....

....

GRATITUDE LIST: *What are you most grateful for today?*

....

....

....

MONTH FOUR

<u>other people</u>

How we relate to other people is immeasurably important. This goes for everyone we come into contact with: family, friends, partners, colleagues, strangers, the waitress at the restaurant, the barista at the coffee shop. How we behave towards other people says far more about us than it ever could about them. The way we treat others can put them down or lift them up, so why not consciously choose to be a glorious ray of sunshine?

Be as kind, compassionate and forgiving as you can possibly be.

Recognise whenever your own insecurities, compulsions, addictions or bad habits push you towards any kind of unhealthy co-dependent behaviour:

• When you people-please: It's not authentic help.
• When you try to exert control over others: It's not authentic help.
• When you try to manipulate people: It's not authentic help.
• When you enable somebody to do something that's bad for them: It's not authentic help.

You must allow other autonomous adults do what it is *they* want to do. Ultimately, if you don't like what another person does, you must put your energy into disengaging from them with dignity. You can't control anybody except yourself and we all need to fundamentally understand and accept that fact with as much love and humility as we can muster. We are 100% accountable for ourselves - and so is everybody else.

Don't expect other people to save you. You must do everything in your power to save yourself. And don't fool yourself into thinking that you can save other people either, because you can't. We are all responsible for our own lives. It's a big enough job just taking care of ourselves. Most of us can't even do that properly half the time. Obviously if you choose to have children, and it <u>should</u> be a considered choice, <u>not</u> a casual consequence, then your life should naturally expand to take care of them too. (Arguably the most important part of raising little ones is to teach them how to take proper care of themselves when they're big.)

If your love life is a disaster because you 'keep picking the wrong ones' don't be so quick to blame the other person and absolve yourself. You are 50% responsible for any relationship you're involved in and 100% responsible for all of your choices. Reclaim your power. Change the trajectory of your life from this moment on. Ask yourself honestly what your true motivations are. Why are you engaging with people who display personality traits that don't suit you? Why are you so eager to get so involved so quickly? Which warning signs are you choosing to overlook? When were you fooled into thinking that you weren't enough on your own?

We all make mistakes. None of us are perfect. We all have sadness and silly stories and regret and remorse in our past. We all want to feel loved and heard and happy. And we all have more power to accomplish that than we tend to assume. You are not the mistakes you have made and you are not destined to repeat them if you don't want to. We each have the freedom to determine our own lives. You can reinvent yourself, any time you want, in any way you want. You don't need permission from anybody but yourself. There are like-minded people all around you, going through the same sort of struggles that you are. Often even worse. Reach out and find them, and if you can, help them without any thought of reward. When we do that, more often than not, we get all the very best rewards without even having to ask and without even realising it. It's a happy hard-earned fact that the healthier you become, the healthier your relationships become with other people.

MONTH .... YEAR ....

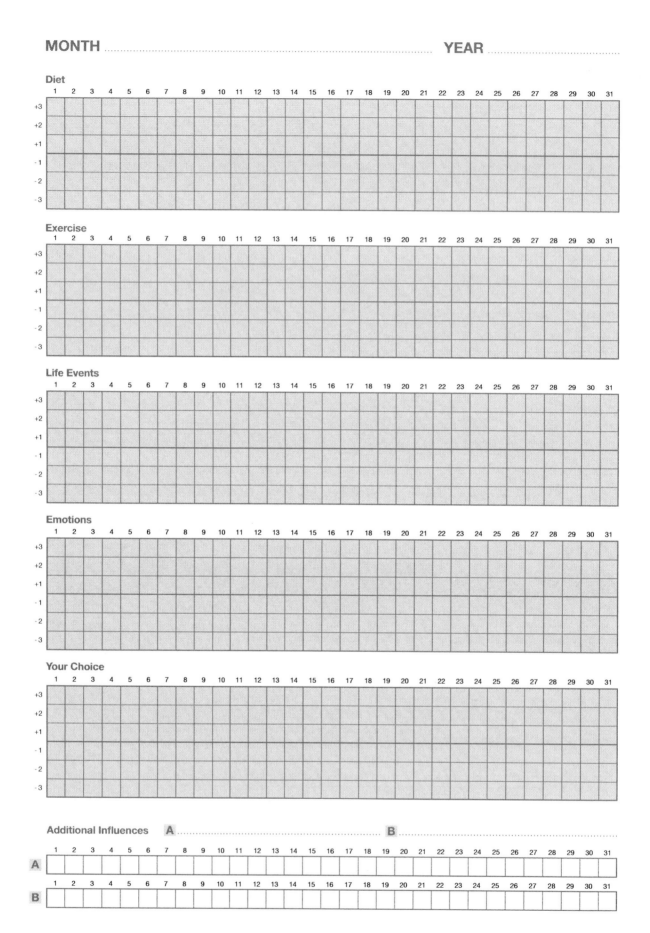

Diet

| | 1 | 2 | 3 | 4 | 5 | 6 | 7 | 8 | 9 | 10 | 11 | 12 | 13 | 14 | 15 | 16 | 17 | 18 | 19 | 20 | 21 | 22 | 23 | 24 | 25 | 26 | 27 | 28 | 29 | 30 | 31 |

+3 +2 +1 -1 -2 -3

Exercise

| | 1 | 2 | 3 | 4 | 5 | 6 | 7 | 8 | 9 | 10 | 11 | 12 | 13 | 14 | 15 | 16 | 17 | 18 | 19 | 20 | 21 | 22 | 23 | 24 | 25 | 26 | 27 | 28 | 29 | 30 | 31 |

+3 +2 +1 -1 -2 -3

Life Events

| | 1 | 2 | 3 | 4 | 5 | 6 | 7 | 8 | 9 | 10 | 11 | 12 | 13 | 14 | 15 | 16 | 17 | 18 | 19 | 20 | 21 | 22 | 23 | 24 | 25 | 26 | 27 | 28 | 29 | 30 | 31 |

+3 +2 +1 -1 -2 -3

Emotions

| | 1 | 2 | 3 | 4 | 5 | 6 | 7 | 8 | 9 | 10 | 11 | 12 | 13 | 14 | 15 | 16 | 17 | 18 | 19 | 20 | 21 | 22 | 23 | 24 | 25 | 26 | 27 | 28 | 29 | 30 | 31 |

+3 +2 +1 -1 -2 -3

Your Choice

| | 1 | 2 | 3 | 4 | 5 | 6 | 7 | 8 | 9 | 10 | 11 | 12 | 13 | 14 | 15 | 16 | 17 | 18 | 19 | 20 | 21 | 22 | 23 | 24 | 25 | 26 | 27 | 28 | 29 | 30 | 31 |

+3 +2 +1 -1 -2 -3

Additional Influences   A ....   B ....

A

B

DATE .... **YEAR** ....

FOOD: *What did you eat today?*

BREAKFAST: ....

Snack: ....

LUNCH: ....

Snack: ....

DINNER: ....

Snack: ....

DRINK: *What did you drink today?*

Any caffeinated drinks: ....

Any alcoholic drinks: ....

Any other drinks: ....

Any other drugs ingested: (including prescription, recreational, over the counter and nicotine) ....

....

QUICK CHECKLIST

WATER - how many litres? ☐   MEDITATION - how many minutes? ☐

SLEEP - how many hours? ☐   EXERCISE - how many minutes? ☐

LIFE EVENTS: *What happened today?*

....

....

....

EMOTIONS/THOUGHTS: *How did you feel today?*

....

....

....

CONCERNS LIST: *What bothered you most today?*

....

....

....

GRATITUDE LIST: *What are you most grateful for today?*

....

....

....

DATE .... **YEAR** ....

FOOD: *What did you eat today?*

BREAKFAST: ....

Snack: ....

LUNCH: ....

Snack: ....

DINNER: ....

Snack: ....

DRINK: *What did you drink today?*

Any caffeinated drinks: ....

Any alcoholic drinks: ....

Any other drinks: ....

Any other drugs ingested: (including prescription, recreational, over the counter and nicotine) ....

....

QUICK CHECKLIST

WATER - how many litres? ▢   MEDITATION - how many minutes? ▢

SLEEP - how many hours? ▢   EXERCISE - how many minutes? ▢

LIFE EVENTS: *What happened today?*

....

....

....

EMOTIONS/THOUGHTS: *How did you feel today?*

....

....

....

CONCERNS LIST: *What bothered you most today?*

....

....

....

GRATITUDE LIST: *What are you most grateful for today?*

....

....

....

DATE .... **YEAR** ....

FOOD: *What did you eat today?*

BREAKFAST: ....

Snack: ....

LUNCH: ....

Snack: ....

DINNER: ....

Snack: ....

DRINK: *What did you drink today?*

Any caffeinated drinks: ....

Any alcoholic drinks: ....

Any other drinks: ....

Any other drugs ingested: (including prescription, recreational, over the counter and nicotine) ....

....

QUICK CHECKLIST

WATER - how many litres? ▢   MEDITATION - how many minutes? ▢

SLEEP - how many hours? ▢   EXERCISE - how many minutes? ▢

LIFE EVENTS: *What happened today?*

....

....

....

EMOTIONS/THOUGHTS: *How did you feel today?*

....

....

....

CONCERNS LIST: *What bothered you most today?*

....

....

....

GRATITUDE LIST: *What are you most grateful for today?*

....

....

....

DATE .... **YEAR** ....

FOOD: *What did you eat today?*

BREAKFAST: ....

Snack: ....

LUNCH: ....

Snack: ....

DINNER: ....

Snack: ....

DRINK: *What did you drink today?*

Any caffeinated drinks: ....

Any alcoholic drinks: ....

Any other drinks: ....

Any other drugs ingested: (including prescription, recreational, over the counter and nicotine) ....

....

QUICK CHECKLIST

WATER - how many litres? ▫   MEDITATION - how many minutes? ▫

SLEEP - how many hours? ▫   EXERCISE - how many minutes? ▫

LIFE EVENTS: *What happened today?*

....

....

....

EMOTIONS/THOUGHTS: *How did you feel today?*

....

....

....

CONCERNS LIST: *What bothered you most today?*

....

....

....

GRATITUDE LIST: *What are you most grateful for today?*

....

....

....

DATE .... **YEAR** ....

FOOD: *What did you eat today?*

BREAKFAST: ....

Snack: ....

LUNCH: ....

Snack: ....

DINNER: ....

Snack: ....

DRINK: *What did you drink today?*

Any caffeinated drinks: ....

Any alcoholic drinks: ....

Any other drinks: ....

Any other drugs ingested: (including prescription, recreational, over the counter and nicotine) ....

....

QUICK CHECKLIST

WATER - how many litres? ▢   MEDITATION - how many minutes? ▢

SLEEP - how many hours? ▢   EXERCISE - how many minutes? ▢

LIFE EVENTS: *What happened today?*

....

....

....

EMOTIONS/THOUGHTS: *How did you feel today?*

....

....

....

CONCERNS LIST: *What bothered you most today?*

....

....

....

GRATITUDE LIST: *What are you most grateful for today?*

....

....

....

DATE .... **YEAR** ....

FOOD: *What did you eat today?*

BREAKFAST: ....

Snack: ....

LUNCH: ....

Snack: ....

DINNER: ....

Snack: ....

DRINK: *What did you drink today?*

Any caffeinated drinks: ....

Any alcoholic drinks: ....

Any other drinks: ....

Any other drugs ingested: (including prescription, recreational, over the counter and nicotine) ....

....

QUICK CHECKLIST

WATER - how many litres? ▢   MEDITATION - how many minutes? ▢

SLEEP - how many hours? ▢   EXERCISE - how many minutes? ▢

LIFE EVENTS: *What happened today?*

....

....

....

EMOTIONS/THOUGHTS: *How did you feel today?*

....

....

....

CONCERNS LIST: *What bothered you most today?*

....

....

....

GRATITUDE LIST: *What are you most grateful for today?*

....

....

....

DATE .... **YEAR** ....

FOOD: *What did you eat today?*

BREAKFAST: ....

Snack: ....

LUNCH: ....

Snack: ....

DINNER: ....

Snack: ....

DRINK: *What did you drink today?*

Any caffeinated drinks: ....

Any alcoholic drinks: ....

Any other drinks: ....

Any other drugs ingested: (including prescription, recreational, over the counter and nicotine) ....

....

QUICK CHECKLIST

WATER - how many litres? ▨   MEDITATION - how many minutes? ▨

SLEEP - how many hours? ▨   EXERCISE - how many minutes? ▨

LIFE EVENTS: *What happened today?*

....

....

....

EMOTIONS/THOUGHTS: *How did you feel today?*

....

....

....

CONCERNS LIST: *What bothered you most today?*

....

....

....

GRATITUDE LIST: *What are you most grateful for today?*

....

....

....

DATE .... **YEAR** ....

FOOD: *What did you eat today?*

BREAKFAST: ....

Snack: ....

LUNCH: ....

Snack: ....

DINNER: ....

Snack: ....

DRINK: *What did you drink today?*

Any caffeinated drinks: ....

Any alcoholic drinks: ....

Any other drinks: ....

Any other drugs ingested: (including prescription, recreational, over the counter and nicotine) ....

....

QUICK CHECKLIST

WATER - how many litres? ▨   MEDITATION - how many minutes? ▨

SLEEP - how many hours? ▨   EXERCISE - how many minutes? ▨

LIFE EVENTS: *What happened today?*

....

....

....

EMOTIONS/THOUGHTS: *How did you feel today?*

....

....

....

CONCERNS LIST: *What bothered you most today?*

....

....

....

GRATITUDE LIST: *What are you most grateful for today?*

....

....

....

DATE .... **YEAR** ....

FOOD: *What did you eat today?*

BREAKFAST: ....

Snack: ....

LUNCH: ....

Snack: ....

DINNER: ....

Snack: ....

DRINK: *What did you drink today?*

Any caffeinated drinks: ....

Any alcoholic drinks: ....

Any other drinks: ....

Any other drugs ingested: (including prescription, recreational, over the counter and nicotine) ....
....

QUICK CHECKLIST

WATER - how many litres? ▢   MEDITATION - how many minutes? ▢

SLEEP - how many hours? ▢   EXERCISE - how many minutes? ▢

LIFE EVENTS: *What happened today?*

....

....

....

EMOTIONS/THOUGHTS: *How did you feel today?*

....

....

....

CONCERNS LIST: *What bothered you most today?*

....

....

....

GRATITUDE LIST: *What are you most grateful for today?*

....

....

....

DATE .... **YEAR** ....

FOOD: *What did you eat today?*

BREAKFAST: ....

Snack: ....

LUNCH: ....

Snack: ....

DINNER: ....

Snack: ....

DRINK: *What did you drink today?*

Any caffeinated drinks: ....

Any alcoholic drinks: ....

Any other drinks: ....

Any other drugs ingested: (including prescription, recreational, over the counter and nicotine) ....

....

QUICK CHECKLIST

WATER - how many litres? ▢   MEDITATION - how many minutes? ▢

SLEEP - how many hours? ▢   EXERCISE - how many minutes? ▢

LIFE EVENTS: *What happened today?*

....

....

....

EMOTIONS/THOUGHTS: *How did you feel today?*

....

....

....

CONCERNS LIST: *What bothered you most today?*

....

....

....

GRATITUDE LIST: *What are you most grateful for today?*

....

....

....

DATE .... **YEAR** ....

FOOD: *What did you eat today?*

BREAKFAST: ....

Snack: ....

LUNCH: ....

Snack: ....

DINNER: ....

Snack: ....

DRINK: *What did you drink today?*

Any caffeinated drinks: ....

Any alcoholic drinks: ....

Any other drinks: ....

Any other drugs ingested: (including prescription, recreational, over the counter and nicotine) ....

....

QUICK CHECKLIST

WATER - how many litres? ☐   MEDITATION - how many minutes? ☐

SLEEP - how many hours? ☐   EXERCISE - how many minutes? ☐

LIFE EVENTS: *What happened today?*

....

....

....

EMOTIONS/THOUGHTS: *How did you feel today?*

....

....

....

CONCERNS LIST: *What bothered you most today?*

....

....

....

GRATITUDE LIST: *What are you most grateful for today?*

....

....

....

DATE .... **YEAR** ....

FOOD: *What did you eat today?*

BREAKFAST: ....

Snack: ....

LUNCH: ....

Snack: ....

DINNER: ....

Snack: ....

DRINK: *What did you drink today?*

Any caffeinated drinks: ....

Any alcoholic drinks: ....

Any other drinks: ....

Any other drugs ingested: (including prescription, recreational, over the counter and nicotine) ....

....

QUICK CHECKLIST

WATER - how many litres? ▢   MEDITATION - how many minutes? ▢

SLEEP - how many hours? ▢   EXERCISE - how many minutes? ▢

LIFE EVENTS: *What happened today?*

....

....

....

EMOTIONS/THOUGHTS: *How did you feel today?*

....

....

....

CONCERNS LIST: *What bothered you most today?*

....

....

....

GRATITUDE LIST: *What are you most grateful for today?*

....

....

....

DATE .... **YEAR** ....

FOOD: *What did you eat today?*

BREAKFAST: ....

Snack: ....

LUNCH: ....

Snack: ....

DINNER: ....

Snack: ....

DRINK: *What did you drink today?*

Any caffeinated drinks: ....

Any alcoholic drinks: ....

Any other drinks: ....

Any other drugs ingested: (including prescription, recreational, over the counter and nicotine) ....

....

QUICK CHECKLIST

WATER - how many litres? ▨   MEDITATION - how many minutes? ▨

SLEEP - how many hours? ▨   EXERCISE - how many minutes? ▨

LIFE EVENTS: *What happened today?*

....

....

....

EMOTIONS/THOUGHTS: *How did you feel today?*

....

....

....

CONCERNS LIST: *What bothered you most today?*

....

....

....

GRATITUDE LIST: *What are you most grateful for today?*

....

....

....

DATE .... **YEAR** ....

FOOD: *What did you eat today?*

BREAKFAST: ....

Snack: ....

LUNCH: ....

Snack: ....

DINNER: ....

Snack: ....

DRINK: *What did you drink today?*

Any caffeinated drinks: ....

Any alcoholic drinks: ....

Any other drinks: ....

Any other drugs ingested: (including prescription, recreational, over the counter and nicotine) ....

....

QUICK CHECKLIST

WATER - how many litres? ☐   MEDITATION - how many minutes? ☐

SLEEP - how many hours? ☐   EXERCISE - how many minutes? ☐

LIFE EVENTS: *What happened today?*

....

....

....

EMOTIONS/THOUGHTS: *How did you feel today?*

....

....

....

CONCERNS LIST: *What bothered you most today?*

....

....

....

GRATITUDE LIST: *What are you most grateful for today?*

....

....

....

DATE .... **YEAR** ....

FOOD: *What did you eat today?*

BREAKFAST: ....

Snack: ....

LUNCH: ....

Snack: ....

DINNER: ....

Snack: ....

DRINK: *What did you drink today?*

Any caffeinated drinks: ....

Any alcoholic drinks: ....

Any other drinks: ....

Any other drugs ingested: (including prescription, recreational, over the counter and nicotine) ....

....

QUICK CHECKLIST

WATER - how many litres? ▢   MEDITATION - how many minutes? ▢

SLEEP - how many hours? ▢   EXERCISE - how many minutes? ▢

LIFE EVENTS: *What happened today?*

....

....

....

EMOTIONS/THOUGHTS: *How did you feel today?*

....

....

....

CONCERNS LIST: *What bothered you most today?*

....

....

....

GRATITUDE LIST: *What are you most grateful for today?*

....

....

....

DATE .... YEAR ....

FOOD: *What did you eat today?*

BREAKFAST: ....

Snack: ....

LUNCH: ....

Snack: ....

DINNER: ....

Snack: ....

DRINK: *What did you drink today?*

Any caffeinated drinks: ....

Any alcoholic drinks: ....

Any other drinks: ....

Any other drugs ingested: (including prescription, recreational, over the counter and nicotine) ....

....

QUICK CHECKLIST

WATER - how many litres? ▢   MEDITATION - how many minutes? ▢

SLEEP - how many hours? ▢   EXERCISE - how many minutes? ▢

LIFE EVENTS: *What happened today?*

....

....

....

EMOTIONS/THOUGHTS: *How did you feel today?*

....

....

....

CONCERNS LIST: *What bothered you most today?*

....

....

....

GRATITUDE LIST: *What are you most grateful for today?*

....

....

....

DATE .... **YEAR** ....

FOOD: *What did you eat today?*

BREAKFAST: ....

Snack: ....

LUNCH: ....

Snack: ....

DINNER: ....

Snack: ....

DRINK: *What did you drink today?*

Any caffeinated drinks: ....

Any alcoholic drinks: ....

Any other drinks: ....

Any other drugs ingested: (including prescription, recreational, over the counter and nicotine) ....

....

QUICK CHECKLIST

WATER - how many litres? ☐   MEDITATION - how many minutes? ☐

SLEEP - how many hours? ☐   EXERCISE - how many minutes? ☐

LIFE EVENTS: *What happened today?*

....

....

....

EMOTIONS/THOUGHTS: *How did you feel today?*

....

....

....

CONCERNS LIST: *What bothered you most today?*

....

....

....

GRATITUDE LIST: *What are you most grateful for today?*

....

....

....

DATE .... YEAR ....

FOOD: *What did you eat today?*

BREAKFAST: ....

Snack: ....

LUNCH: ....

Snack: ....

DINNER: ....

Snack: ....

DRINK: *What did you drink today?*

Any caffeinated drinks: ....

Any alcoholic drinks: ....

Any other drinks: ....

Any other drugs ingested: (including prescription, recreational, over the counter and nicotine) ....
....

QUICK CHECKLIST

WATER - how many litres?   ▨   MEDITATION - how many minutes? ▨

SLEEP - how many hours?   ▨   EXERCISE - how many minutes?   ▨

LIFE EVENTS: *What happened today?*

....
....
....

EMOTIONS/THOUGHTS: *How did you feel today?*

....
....
....

CONCERNS LIST: *What bothered you most today?*

....
....
....

GRATITUDE LIST: *What are you most grateful for today?*

....
....
....

DATE .... **YEAR** ....

FOOD: *What did you eat today?*

BREAKFAST: ....

Snack: ....

LUNCH: ....

Snack: ....

DINNER: ....

Snack: ....

DRINK: *What did you drink today?*

Any caffeinated drinks: ....

Any alcoholic drinks: ....

Any other drinks: ....

Any other drugs ingested: (including prescription, recreational, over the counter and nicotine) ....

....

QUICK CHECKLIST

WATER - how many litres?　▢　　MEDITATION - how many minutes?　▢

SLEEP - how many hours?　▢　　EXERCISE - how many minutes?　▢

LIFE EVENTS: *What happened today?*

....

....

....

EMOTIONS/THOUGHTS: *How did you feel today?*

....

....

....

CONCERNS LIST: *What bothered you most today?*

....

....

....

GRATITUDE LIST: *What are you most grateful for today?*

....

....

....

DATE .... **YEAR** ....

FOOD: *What did you eat today?*

BREAKFAST: ....

Snack: ....

LUNCH: ....

Snack: ....

DINNER: ....

Snack: ....

DRINK: *What did you drink today?*

Any caffeinated drinks: ....

Any alcoholic drinks: ....

Any other drinks: ....

Any other drugs ingested: (including prescription, recreational, over the counter and nicotine) ....

....

QUICK CHECKLIST

WATER - how many litres? ▨   MEDITATION - how many minutes? ▨

SLEEP - how many hours? ▨   EXERCISE - how many minutes? ▨

LIFE EVENTS: *What happened today?*

....

....

....

EMOTIONS/THOUGHTS: *How did you feel today?*

....

....

....

CONCERNS LIST: *What bothered you most today?*

....

....

....

GRATITUDE LIST: *What are you most grateful for today?*

....

....

....

DATE .... **YEAR** ....

FOOD: *What did you eat today?*

BREAKFAST: ....

Snack: ....

LUNCH: ....

Snack: ....

DINNER: ....

Snack: ....

DRINK: *What did you drink today?*

Any caffeinated drinks: ....

Any alcoholic drinks: ....

Any other drinks: ....

Any other drugs ingested: (including prescription, recreational, over the counter and nicotine) ....

....

QUICK CHECKLIST

WATER - how many litres? ▨   MEDITATION - how many minutes? ▨

SLEEP - how many hours? ▨   EXERCISE - how many minutes? ▨

LIFE EVENTS: *What happened today?*

....

....

....

EMOTIONS/THOUGHTS: *How did you feel today?*

....

....

....

CONCERNS LIST: *What bothered you most today?*

....

....

....

GRATITUDE LIST: *What are you most grateful for today?*

....

....

....

DATE .... **YEAR** ....

FOOD: *What did you eat today?*

BREAKFAST: ....

Snack: ....

LUNCH: ....

Snack: ....

DINNER: ....

Snack: ....

DRINK: *What did you drink today?*

Any caffeinated drinks: ....

Any alcoholic drinks: ....

Any other drinks: ....

Any other drugs ingested: (including prescription, recreational, over the counter and nicotine) ....

....

QUICK CHECKLIST

WATER - how many litres?   ☐   MEDITATION - how many minutes?   ☐

SLEEP - how many hours?   ☐   EXERCISE - how many minutes?   ☐

LIFE EVENTS: *What happened today?*

....

....

....

EMOTIONS/THOUGHTS: *How did you feel today?*

....

....

....

CONCERNS LIST: *What bothered you most today?*

....

....

....

GRATITUDE LIST: *What are you most grateful for today?*

....

....

....

DATE .... **YEAR** ....

FOOD: *What did you eat today?*

BREAKFAST: ....

Snack: ....

LUNCH: ....

Snack: ....

DINNER: ....

Snack: ....

DRINK: *What did you drink today?*

Any caffeinated drinks: ....

Any alcoholic drinks: ....

Any other drinks: ....

Any other drugs ingested: (including prescription, recreational, over the counter and nicotine) ....

....

QUICK CHECKLIST

WATER - how many litres? ▢   MEDITATION - how many minutes? ▢

SLEEP - how many hours? ▢   EXERCISE - how many minutes? ▢

LIFE EVENTS: *What happened today?*

....

....

....

EMOTIONS/THOUGHTS: *How did you feel today?*

....

....

....

CONCERNS LIST: *What bothered you most today?*

....

....

....

GRATITUDE LIST: *What are you most grateful for today?*

....

....

....

DATE .... **YEAR** ....

FOOD: *What did you eat today?*

BREAKFAST: ....

Snack: ....

LUNCH: ....

Snack: ....

DINNER: ....

Snack: ....

DRINK: *What did you drink today?*

Any caffeinated drinks: ....

Any alcoholic drinks: ....

Any other drinks: ....

Any other drugs ingested: (including prescription, recreational, over the counter and nicotine) ....

....

QUICK CHECKLIST

WATER - how many litres? ☐   MEDITATION - how many minutes? ☐

SLEEP - how many hours? ☐   EXERCISE - how many minutes? ☐

LIFE EVENTS: *What happened today?*

....

....

....

EMOTIONS/THOUGHTS: *How did you feel today?*

....

....

....

CONCERNS LIST: *What bothered you most today?*

....

....

....

GRATITUDE LIST: *What are you most grateful for today?*

....

....

....

DATE .... **YEAR** ....

FOOD: *What did you eat today?*

BREAKFAST: ....

Snack: ....

LUNCH: ....

Snack: ....

DINNER: ....

Snack: ....

DRINK: *What did you drink today?*

Any caffeinated drinks: ....

Any alcoholic drinks: ....

Any other drinks: ....

Any other drugs ingested: (including prescription, recreational, over the counter and nicotine) ....

....

QUICK CHECKLIST

WATER - how many litres?　▢　　MEDITATION - how many minutes?　▢

SLEEP - how many hours?　▢　　EXERCISE - how many minutes?　▢

LIFE EVENTS: *What happened today?*

....

....

....

EMOTIONS/THOUGHTS: *How did you feel today?*

....

....

....

CONCERNS LIST: *What bothered you most today?*

....

....

....

GRATITUDE LIST: *What are you most grateful for today?*

....

....

....

DATE .... **YEAR** ....

FOOD: *What did you eat today?*

BREAKFAST: ....

Snack: ....

LUNCH: ....

Snack: ....

DINNER: ....

Snack: ....

DRINK: *What did you drink today?*

Any caffeinated drinks: ....

Any alcoholic drinks: ....

Any other drinks: ....

Any other drugs ingested: (including prescription, recreational, over the counter and nicotine) ....

....

QUICK CHECKLIST

WATER - how many litres? ▢   MEDITATION - how many minutes? ▢

SLEEP - how many hours? ▢   EXERCISE - how many minutes? ▢

LIFE EVENTS: *What happened today?*

....

....

....

EMOTIONS/THOUGHTS: *How did you feel today?*

....

....

....

CONCERNS LIST: *What bothered you most today?*

....

....

....

GRATITUDE LIST: *What are you most grateful for today?*

....

....

....

DATE .... **YEAR** ....

FOOD: *What did you eat today?*

BREAKFAST: ....

Snack: ....

LUNCH: ....

Snack: ....

DINNER: ....

Snack: ....

DRINK: *What did you drink today?*

Any caffeinated drinks: ....

Any alcoholic drinks: ....

Any other drinks: ....

Any other drugs ingested: (including prescription, recreational, over the counter and nicotine) ....

....

QUICK CHECKLIST

WATER - how many litres? ☐   MEDITATION - how many minutes? ☐

SLEEP - how many hours? ☐   EXERCISE - how many minutes? ☐

LIFE EVENTS: *What happened today?*

....

....

....

EMOTIONS/THOUGHTS: *How did you feel today?*

....

....

....

CONCERNS LIST: *What bothered you most today?*

....

....

....

GRATITUDE LIST: *What are you most grateful for today?*

....

....

....

DATE .... **YEAR** ....

FOOD: *What did you eat today?*

BREAKFAST: ....

Snack: ....

LUNCH: ....

Snack: ....

DINNER: ....

Snack: ....

DRINK: *What did you drink today?*

Any caffeinated drinks: ....

Any alcoholic drinks: ....

Any other drinks: ....

Any other drugs ingested: (including prescription, recreational, over the counter and nicotine) ....

....

QUICK CHECKLIST

WATER - how many litres? ☐   MEDITATION - how many minutes? ☐

SLEEP - how many hours? ☐   EXERCISE - how many minutes? ☐

LIFE EVENTS: *What happened today?*

....

....

....

EMOTIONS/THOUGHTS: *How did you feel today?*

....

....

....

CONCERNS LIST: *What bothered you most today?*

....

....

....

GRATITUDE LIST: *What are you most grateful for today?*

....

....

....

DATE .... **YEAR** ....

FOOD: *What did you eat today?*

BREAKFAST: ....

Snack: ....

LUNCH: ....

Snack: ....

DINNER: ....

Snack: ....

DRINK: *What did you drink today?*

Any caffeinated drinks: ....

Any alcoholic drinks: ....

Any other drinks: ....

Any other drugs ingested: (including prescription, recreational, over the counter and nicotine) ....

....

QUICK CHECKLIST

WATER - how many litres? ▨   MEDITATION - how many minutes? ▨

SLEEP - how many hours? ▨   EXERCISE - how many minutes? ▨

LIFE EVENTS: *What happened today?*

....

....

....

EMOTIONS/THOUGHTS: *How did you feel today?*

....

....

....

CONCERNS LIST: *What bothered you most today?*

....

....

....

GRATITUDE LIST: *What are you most grateful for today?*

....

....

....

DATE .... **YEAR** ....

FOOD: *What did you eat today?*

BREAKFAST: ....

Snack: ....

LUNCH: ....

Snack: ....

DINNER: ....

Snack: ....

DRINK: *What did you drink today?*

Any caffeinated drinks: ....

Any alcoholic drinks: ....

Any other drinks: ....

Any other drugs ingested: (including prescription, recreational, over the counter and nicotine) ....

....

QUICK CHECKLIST

WATER - how many litres? ▨   MEDITATION - how many minutes? ▨

SLEEP - how many hours? ▨   EXERCISE - how many minutes? ▨

LIFE EVENTS: *What happened today?*

....

....

....

EMOTIONS/THOUGHTS: *How did you feel today?*

....

....

....

CONCERNS LIST: *What bothered you most today?*

....

....

....

GRATITUDE LIST: *What are you most grateful for today?*

....

....

....

DATE .... **YEAR** ....

FOOD: *What did you eat today?*

BREAKFAST: ....

Snack: ....

LUNCH: ....

Snack: ....

DINNER: ....

Snack: ....

DRINK: *What did you drink today?*

Any caffeinated drinks: ....

Any alcoholic drinks: ....

Any other drinks: ....

Any other drugs ingested: (including prescription, recreational, over the counter and nicotine) ....

....

QUICK CHECKLIST

WATER - how many litres? ▢   MEDITATION - how many minutes? ▢

SLEEP - how many hours? ▢   EXERCISE - how many minutes? ▢

LIFE EVENTS: *What happened today?*

....

....

....

EMOTIONS/THOUGHTS: *How did you feel today?*

....

....

....

CONCERNS LIST: *What bothered you most today?*

....

....

....

GRATITUDE LIST: *What are you most grateful for today?*

....

....

....

MONTH

FIVE

<u>honesty and accountability</u>

To get the best results out of The Off The Rocks Journal, it is absolutely imperative that you are completely honest with yourself. You will only see genuine results and progress if you record genuine information.

We must all strive to take honest responsibility for our own actions in life. We all get off track from time to time in one area or another, but you can decide to reclaim control of your life again any time you like and The Off The Rocks Journal will help you to do this. No-one else can do this for you. You are 100% accountable for your own life (and so is everybody else for theirs). The first step towards self-empowerment and improving your life is to be totally, completely, unashamedly honest with yourself.

Where are you justifying your own bad behaviour? Where are you turning a blind eye? Where are you sabotaging yourself? What are your strengths? What are your weaknesses? What are you goals? What are you proud of? What are you ashamed of? You won't find the genuine answers to any of these questions unless you are truthful with yourself.

It's time to drop the excuses that have held you back until now and realise that you can do things differently if you really want to. Your future will depend on the decisions you make today. You are capable of much more than you realise and the journey towards your new improved life is yours for the taking.

You are always just one decision away from a completely different outcome.

MONTH .... YEAR ....

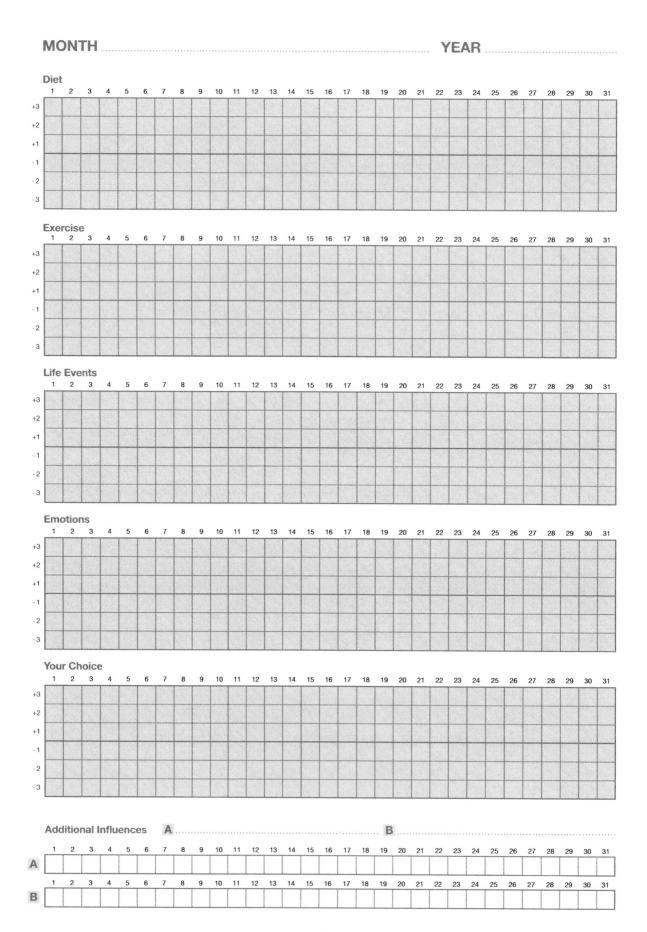

Diet

Exercise

Life Events

Emotions

Your Choice

Additional Influences   A .... B ....

DATE .... **YEAR** ....

FOOD: *What did you eat today?*

BREAKFAST: ....

Snack: ....

LUNCH: ....

Snack: ....

DINNER: ....

Snack: ....

DRINK: *What did you drink today?*

Any caffeinated drinks: ....

Any alcoholic drinks: ....

Any other drinks: ....

Any other drugs ingested: (including prescription, recreational, over the counter and nicotine) ....

....

QUICK CHECKLIST

WATER - how many litres? ☐   MEDITATION - how many minutes? ☐

SLEEP - how many hours? ☐   EXERCISE - how many minutes? ☐

LIFE EVENTS: *What happened today?*

....

....

....

EMOTIONS/THOUGHTS: *How did you feel today?*

....

....

....

CONCERNS LIST: *What bothered you most today?*

....

....

....

GRATITUDE LIST: *What are you most grateful for today?*

....

....

....

DATE .... **YEAR** ....

FOOD: *What did you eat today?*

BREAKFAST: ....

Snack: ....

LUNCH: ....

Snack: ....

DINNER: ....

Snack: ....

DRINK: *What did you drink today?*

Any caffeinated drinks: ....

Any alcoholic drinks: ....

Any other drinks: ....

Any other drugs ingested: (including prescription, recreational, over the counter and nicotine) ....

....

QUICK CHECKLIST

WATER - how many litres? ☐   MEDITATION - how many minutes? ☐

SLEEP - how many hours? ☐   EXERCISE - how many minutes? ☐

LIFE EVENTS: *What happened today?*

....

....

....

EMOTIONS/THOUGHTS: *How did you feel today?*

....

....

....

CONCERNS LIST: *What bothered you most today?*

....

....

....

GRATITUDE LIST: *What are you most grateful for today?*

....

....

....

DATE .... **YEAR** ....

FOOD: *What did you eat today?*

BREAKFAST: ....

Snack: ....

LUNCH: ....

Snack: ....

DINNER: ....

Snack: ....

DRINK: *What did you drink today?*

Any caffeinated drinks: ....

Any alcoholic drinks: ....

Any other drinks: ....

Any other drugs ingested: (including prescription, recreational, over the counter and nicotine) ....

....

QUICK CHECKLIST

WATER - how many litres? ▨   MEDITATION - how many minutes? ▨

SLEEP - how many hours? ▨   EXERCISE - how many minutes? ▨

LIFE EVENTS: *What happened today?*

....

....

....

EMOTIONS/THOUGHTS: *How did you feel today?*

....

....

....

CONCERNS LIST: *What bothered you most today?*

....

....

....

GRATITUDE LIST: *What are you most grateful for today?*

....

....

....

DATE .... **YEAR** ....

FOOD: *What did you eat today?*

BREAKFAST: ....

Snack: ....

LUNCH: ....

Snack: ....

DINNER: ....

Snack: ....

DRINK: *What did you drink today?*

Any caffeinated drinks: ....

Any alcoholic drinks: ....

Any other drinks: ....

Any other drugs ingested: (including prescription, recreational, over the counter and nicotine) ....

....

QUICK CHECKLIST

WATER - how many litres? ▢   MEDITATION - how many minutes? ▢

SLEEP - how many hours? ▢   EXERCISE - how many minutes? ▢

LIFE EVENTS: *What happened today?*

....

....

....

EMOTIONS/THOUGHTS: *How did you feel today?*

....

....

....

CONCERNS LIST: *What bothered you most today?*

....

....

....

GRATITUDE LIST: *What are you most grateful for today?*

....

....

....

DATE .... **YEAR** ....

FOOD: *What did you eat today?*

BREAKFAST: ....

Snack: ....

LUNCH: ....

Snack: ....

DINNER: ....

Snack: ....

DRINK: *What did you drink today?*

Any caffeinated drinks: ....

Any alcoholic drinks: ....

Any other drinks: ....

Any other drugs ingested: (including prescription, recreational, over the counter and nicotine) ....

....

QUICK CHECKLIST

WATER - how many litres? ▨   MEDITATION - how many minutes? ▨

SLEEP - how many hours? ▨   EXERCISE - how many minutes? ▨

LIFE EVENTS: *What happened today?*

....

....

....

EMOTIONS/THOUGHTS: *How did you feel today?*

....

....

....

CONCERNS LIST: *What bothered you most today?*

....

....

....

GRATITUDE LIST: *What are you most grateful for today?*

....

....

....

DATE .... **YEAR** ....

FOOD: *What did you eat today?*

BREAKFAST: ....

Snack: ....

LUNCH: ....

Snack: ....

DINNER: ....

Snack: ....

DRINK: *What did you drink today?*

Any caffeinated drinks: ....

Any alcoholic drinks: ....

Any other drinks: ....

Any other drugs ingested: (including prescription, recreational, over the counter and nicotine) ....

....

QUICK CHECKLIST

WATER - how many litres? ▢   MEDITATION - how many minutes? ▢

SLEEP - how many hours? ▢   EXERCISE - how many minutes? ▢

LIFE EVENTS: *What happened today?*

....

....

....

EMOTIONS/THOUGHTS: *How did you feel today?*

....

....

....

CONCERNS LIST: *What bothered you most today?*

....

....

....

GRATITUDE LIST: *What are you most grateful for today?*

....

....

....

DATE .... **YEAR** ....

FOOD: *What did you eat today?*

BREAKFAST: ....

Snack: ....

LUNCH: ....

Snack: ....

DINNER: ....

Snack: ....

DRINK: *What did you drink today?*

Any caffeinated drinks: ....

Any alcoholic drinks: ....

Any other drinks: ....

Any other drugs ingested: (including prescription, recreational, over the counter and nicotine) ....

....

QUICK CHECKLIST

WATER - how many litres? ▨   MEDITATION - how many minutes? ▨

SLEEP - how many hours? ▨   EXERCISE - how many minutes? ▨

LIFE EVENTS: *What happened today?*

....

....

....

EMOTIONS/THOUGHTS: *How did you feel today?*

....

....

....

CONCERNS LIST: *What bothered you most today?*

....

....

....

GRATITUDE LIST: *What are you most grateful for today?*

....

....

....

DATE .... **YEAR** ....

FOOD: *What did you eat today?*

BREAKFAST: ....

Snack: ....

LUNCH: ....

Snack: ....

DINNER: ....

Snack: ....

DRINK: *What did you drink today?*

Any caffeinated drinks: ....

Any alcoholic drinks: ....

Any other drinks: ....

Any other drugs ingested: (including prescription, recreational, over the counter and nicotine) ....

....

QUICK CHECKLIST

WATER - how many litres? ☐   MEDITATION - how many minutes? ☐

SLEEP - how many hours? ☐   EXERCISE - how many minutes? ☐

LIFE EVENTS: *What happened today?*

....

....

....

EMOTIONS/THOUGHTS: *How did you feel today?*

....

....

....

CONCERNS LIST: *What bothered you most today?*

....

....

....

GRATITUDE LIST: *What are you most grateful for today?*

....

....

....

DATE .... **YEAR** ....

FOOD: *What did you eat today?*

BREAKFAST: ....

Snack: ....

LUNCH: ....

Snack: ....

DINNER: ....

Snack: ....

DRINK: *What did you drink today?*

Any caffeinated drinks: ....

Any alcoholic drinks: ....

Any other drinks: ....

Any other drugs ingested: (including prescription, recreational, over the counter and nicotine) ....

....

QUICK CHECKLIST

WATER - how many litres? ▨   MEDITATION - how many minutes? ▨

SLEEP - how many hours? ▨   EXERCISE - how many minutes? ▨

LIFE EVENTS: *What happened today?*

....

....

....

EMOTIONS/THOUGHTS: *How did you feel today?*

....

....

....

CONCERNS LIST: *What bothered you most today?*

....

....

....

GRATITUDE LIST: *What are you most grateful for today?*

....

....

....

DATE .... **YEAR** ....

FOOD: *What did you eat today?*

BREAKFAST: ....

Snack: ....

LUNCH: ....

Snack: ....

DINNER: ....

Snack: ....

DRINK: *What did you drink today?*

Any caffeinated drinks: ....

Any alcoholic drinks: ....

Any other drinks: ....

Any other drugs ingested: (including prescription, recreational, over the counter and nicotine) ....

....

QUICK CHECKLIST

WATER - how many litres? ▢   MEDITATION - how many minutes? ▢

SLEEP - how many hours? ▢   EXERCISE - how many minutes? ▢

LIFE EVENTS: *What happened today?*

....

....

....

EMOTIONS/THOUGHTS: *How did you feel today?*

....

....

....

CONCERNS LIST: *What bothered you most today?*

....

....

....

GRATITUDE LIST: *What are you most grateful for today?*

....

....

....

DATE .... **YEAR** ....

FOOD: *What did you eat today?*

BREAKFAST: ....

Snack: ....

LUNCH: ....

Snack: ....

DINNER: ....

Snack: ....

DRINK: *What did you drink today?*

Any caffeinated drinks: ....

Any alcoholic drinks: ....

Any other drinks: ....

Any other drugs ingested: (including prescription, recreational, over the counter and nicotine) ....

....

QUICK CHECKLIST

WATER - how many litres? ▨   MEDITATION - how many minutes? ▨

SLEEP - how many hours? ▨   EXERCISE - how many minutes? ▨

LIFE EVENTS: *What happened today?*

....

....

....

EMOTIONS/THOUGHTS: *How did you feel today?*

....

....

....

CONCERNS LIST: *What bothered you most today?*

....

....

....

GRATITUDE LIST: *What are you most grateful for today?*

....

....

....

DATE .... **YEAR** ....

FOOD: *What did you eat today?*

BREAKFAST: ....

Snack: ....

LUNCH: ....

Snack: ....

DINNER: ....

Snack: ....

DRINK: *What did you drink today?*

Any caffeinated drinks: ....

Any alcoholic drinks: ....

Any other drinks: ....

Any other drugs ingested: (including prescription, recreational, over the counter and nicotine) ....

....

QUICK CHECKLIST

WATER - how many litres? ☐   MEDITATION - how many minutes? ☐

SLEEP - how many hours? ☐   EXERCISE - how many minutes? ☐

LIFE EVENTS: *What happened today?*

....

....

....

EMOTIONS/THOUGHTS: *How did you feel today?*

....

....

....

CONCERNS LIST: *What bothered you most today?*

....

....

....

GRATITUDE LIST: *What are you most grateful for today?*

....

....

....

DATE .... **YEAR** ....

FOOD: *What did you eat today?*

BREAKFAST: ....

Snack: ....

LUNCH: ....

Snack: ....

DINNER: ....

Snack: ....

DRINK: *What did you drink today?*

Any caffeinated drinks: ....

Any alcoholic drinks: ....

Any other drinks: ....

Any other drugs ingested: (including prescription, recreational, over the counter and nicotine) ....

....

QUICK CHECKLIST

WATER - how many litres? ☐   MEDITATION - how many minutes? ☐

SLEEP - how many hours? ☐   EXERCISE - how many minutes? ☐

LIFE EVENTS: *What happened today?*

....

....

....

EMOTIONS/THOUGHTS: *How did you feel today?*

....

....

....

CONCERNS LIST: *What bothered you most today?*

....

....

....

GRATITUDE LIST: *What are you most grateful for today?*

....

....

....

DATE .... **YEAR** ....

FOOD: *What did you eat today?*

BREAKFAST: ....

Snack: ....

LUNCH: ....

Snack: ....

DINNER: ....

Snack: ....

DRINK: *What did you drink today?*

Any caffeinated drinks: ....

Any alcoholic drinks: ....

Any other drinks: ....

Any other drugs ingested: (including prescription, recreational, over the counter and nicotine) ....

....

QUICK CHECKLIST

WATER - how many litres? ☐   MEDITATION - how many minutes? ☐

SLEEP - how many hours? ☐   EXERCISE - how many minutes? ☐

LIFE EVENTS: *What happened today?*

....

....

....

EMOTIONS/THOUGHTS: *How did you feel today?*

....

....

....

CONCERNS LIST: *What bothered you most today?*

....

....

....

GRATITUDE LIST: *What are you most grateful for today?*

....

....

....

DATE .... **YEAR** ....

FOOD: *What did you eat today?*

BREAKFAST: ....

Snack: ....

LUNCH: ....

Snack: ....

DINNER: ....

Snack: ....

DRINK: *What did you drink today?*

Any caffeinated drinks: ....

Any alcoholic drinks: ....

Any other drinks: ....

Any other drugs ingested: (including prescription, recreational, over the counter and nicotine) ....

....

QUICK CHECKLIST

WATER - how many litres? ▨   MEDITATION - how many minutes? ▨

SLEEP - how many hours? ▨   EXERCISE - how many minutes? ▨

LIFE EVENTS: *What happened today?*

....

....

....

EMOTIONS/THOUGHTS: *How did you feel today?*

....

....

....

CONCERNS LIST: *What bothered you most today?*

....

....

....

GRATITUDE LIST: *What are you most grateful for today?*

....

....

....

DATE .... YEAR ....

FOOD: *What did you eat today?*

BREAKFAST: ....

Snack: ....

LUNCH: ....

Snack: ....

DINNER: ....

Snack: ....

DRINK: *What did you drink today?*

Any caffeinated drinks: ....

Any alcoholic drinks: ....

Any other drinks: ....

Any other drugs ingested: (including prescription, recreational, over the counter and nicotine) ....

....

QUICK CHECKLIST

WATER - how many litres? ▢   MEDITATION - how many minutes? ▢

SLEEP - how many hours? ▢   EXERCISE - how many minutes? ▢

LIFE EVENTS: *What happened today?*

....

....

....

EMOTIONS/THOUGHTS: *How did you feel today?*

....

....

....

CONCERNS LIST: *What bothered you most today?*

....

....

....

GRATITUDE LIST: *What are you most grateful for today?*

....

....

....

DATE .... **YEAR** ....

FOOD: *What did you eat today?*

BREAKFAST: ....

Snack: ....

LUNCH: ....

Snack: ....

DINNER: ....

Snack: ....

DRINK: *What did you drink today?*

Any caffeinated drinks: ....

Any alcoholic drinks: ....

Any other drinks: ....

Any other drugs ingested: (including prescription, recreational, over the counter and nicotine) ....

....

QUICK CHECKLIST

WATER - how many litres? ▨   MEDITATION - how many minutes? ▨

SLEEP - how many hours? ▨   EXERCISE - how many minutes? ▨

LIFE EVENTS: *What happened today?*

....

....

....

EMOTIONS/THOUGHTS: *How did you feel today?*

....

....

....

CONCERNS LIST: *What bothered you most today?*

....

....

....

GRATITUDE LIST: *What are you most grateful for today?*

....

....

....

DATE .... **YEAR** ....

FOOD: *What did you eat today?*

BREAKFAST: ....

Snack: ....

LUNCH: ....

Snack: ....

DINNER: ....

Snack: ....

DRINK: *What did you drink today?*

Any caffeinated drinks: ....

Any alcoholic drinks: ....

Any other drinks: ....

Any other drugs ingested: (including prescription, recreational, over the counter and nicotine) ....

....

QUICK CHECKLIST

WATER - how many litres? ☐   MEDITATION - how many minutes? ☐

SLEEP - how many hours? ☐   EXERCISE - how many minutes? ☐

LIFE EVENTS: *What happened today?*

....

....

....

EMOTIONS/THOUGHTS: *How did you feel today?*

....

....

....

CONCERNS LIST: *What bothered you most today?*

....

....

....

GRATITUDE LIST: *What are you most grateful for today?*

....

....

....

DATE .... **YEAR** ....

FOOD: *What did you eat today?*

BREAKFAST: ....

Snack: ....

LUNCH: ....

Snack: ....

DINNER: ....

Snack: ....

DRINK: *What did you drink today?*

Any caffeinated drinks: ....

Any alcoholic drinks: ....

Any other drinks: ....

Any other drugs ingested: (including prescription, recreational, over the counter and nicotine) ....

....

QUICK CHECKLIST

WATER - how many litres? ▨   MEDITATION - how many minutes? ▨

SLEEP - how many hours? ▨   EXERCISE - how many minutes? ▨

LIFE EVENTS: *What happened today?*

....

....

....

EMOTIONS/THOUGHTS: *How did you feel today?*

....

....

....

CONCERNS LIST: *What bothered you most today?*

....

....

....

GRATITUDE LIST: *What are you most grateful for today?*

....

....

....

DATE .... **YEAR** ....

FOOD: *What did you eat today?*

BREAKFAST: ....

Snack: ....

LUNCH: ....

Snack: ....

DINNER: ....

Snack: ....

DRINK: *What did you drink today?*

Any caffeinated drinks: ....

Any alcoholic drinks: ....

Any other drinks: ....

Any other drugs ingested: (including prescription, recreational, over the counter and nicotine) ....

....

QUICK CHECKLIST

WATER - how many litres? ▢   MEDITATION - how many minutes? ▢

SLEEP - how many hours? ▢   EXERCISE - how many minutes? ▢

LIFE EVENTS: *What happened today?*

....

....

....

EMOTIONS/THOUGHTS: *How did you feel today?*

....

....

....

CONCERNS LIST: *What bothered you most today?*

....

....

....

GRATITUDE LIST: *What are you most grateful for today?*

....

....

....

DATE .... **YEAR** ....

FOOD: *What did you eat today?*

BREAKFAST: ....

Snack: ....

LUNCH: ....

Snack: ....

DINNER: ....

Snack: ....

DRINK: *What did you drink today?*

Any caffeinated drinks: ....

Any alcoholic drinks: ....

Any other drinks: ....

Any other drugs ingested: (including prescription, recreational, over the counter and nicotine) ....

....

QUICK CHECKLIST

WATER - how many litres? ▢   MEDITATION - how many minutes? ▢

SLEEP - how many hours? ▢   EXERCISE - how many minutes? ▢

LIFE EVENTS: *What happened today?*

....

....

....

EMOTIONS/THOUGHTS: *How did you feel today?*

....

....

....

CONCERNS LIST: *What bothered you most today?*

....

....

....

GRATITUDE LIST: *What are you most grateful for today?*

....

....

....

DATE .... **YEAR** ....

FOOD: *What did you eat today?*

BREAKFAST: ....

Snack: ....

LUNCH: ....

Snack: ....

DINNER: ....

Snack: ....

DRINK: *What did you drink today?*

Any caffeinated drinks: ....

Any alcoholic drinks: ....

Any other drinks: ....

Any other drugs ingested: (including prescription, recreational, over the counter and nicotine) ....

....

QUICK CHECKLIST

WATER - how many litres? ☐   MEDITATION - how many minutes? ☐

SLEEP - how many hours? ☐   EXERCISE - how many minutes? ☐

LIFE EVENTS: *What happened today?*

....

....

....

EMOTIONS/THOUGHTS: *How did you feel today?*

....

....

....

CONCERNS LIST: *What bothered you most today?*

....

....

....

GRATITUDE LIST: *What are you most grateful for today?*

....

....

....

DATE .... **YEAR** ....

FOOD: *What did you eat today?*

BREAKFAST: ....

Snack: ....

LUNCH: ....

Snack: ....

DINNER: ....

Snack: ....

DRINK: *What did you drink today?*

Any caffeinated drinks: ....

Any alcoholic drinks: ....

Any other drinks: ....

Any other drugs ingested: (including prescription, recreational, over the counter and nicotine) ....

....

QUICK CHECKLIST

WATER - how many litres? ▢   MEDITATION - how many minutes? ▢

SLEEP - how many hours? ▢   EXERCISE - how many minutes? ▢

LIFE EVENTS: *What happened today?*

....

....

....

EMOTIONS/THOUGHTS: *How did you feel today?*

....

....

....

CONCERNS LIST: *What bothered you most today?*

....

....

....

GRATITUDE LIST: *What are you most grateful for today?*

....

....

....

DATE .... **YEAR** ....

FOOD: *What did you eat today?*

BREAKFAST: ....

Snack: ....

LUNCH: ....

Snack: ....

DINNER: ....

Snack: ....

DRINK: *What did you drink today?*

Any caffeinated drinks: ....

Any alcoholic drinks: ....

Any other drinks: ....

Any other drugs ingested: (including prescription, recreational, over the counter and nicotine) ....

....

QUICK CHECKLIST

WATER - how many litres? ▦   MEDITATION - how many minutes? ▦

SLEEP - how many hours? ▦   EXERCISE - how many minutes? ▦

LIFE EVENTS: *What happened today?*

....

....

....

EMOTIONS/THOUGHTS: *How did you feel today?*

....

....

....

CONCERNS LIST: *What bothered you most today?*

....

....

....

GRATITUDE LIST: *What are you most grateful for today?*

....

....

....

DATE .... **YEAR** ....

FOOD: *What did you eat today?*

BREAKFAST: ....

Snack: ....

LUNCH: ....

Snack: ....

DINNER: ....

Snack: ....

DRINK: *What did you drink today?*

Any caffeinated drinks: ....

Any alcoholic drinks: ....

Any other drinks: ....

Any other drugs ingested: (including prescription, recreational, over the counter and nicotine) ....

....

QUICK CHECKLIST

WATER - how many litres? ☐   MEDITATION - how many minutes? ☐

SLEEP - how many hours? ☐   EXERCISE - how many minutes? ☐

LIFE EVENTS: *What happened today?*

....

....

....

EMOTIONS/THOUGHTS: *How did you feel today?*

....

....

....

CONCERNS LIST: *What bothered you most today?*

....

....

....

GRATITUDE LIST: *What are you most grateful for today?*

....

....

....

DATE .... YEAR ....

FOOD: *What did you eat today?*

BREAKFAST: ....

Snack: ....

LUNCH: ....

Snack: ....

DINNER: ....

Snack: ....

DRINK: *What did you drink today?*

Any caffeinated drinks: ....

Any alcoholic drinks: ....

Any other drinks: ....

Any other drugs ingested: (including prescription, recreational, over the counter and nicotine) ....

QUICK CHECKLIST

WATER - how many litres? ☐   MEDITATION - how many minutes? ☐

SLEEP - how many hours? ☐   EXERCISE - how many minutes? ☐

LIFE EVENTS: *What happened today?*

....

....

....

EMOTIONS/THOUGHTS: *How did you feel today?*

....

....

....

CONCERNS LIST: *What bothered you most today?*

....

....

....

GRATITUDE LIST: *What are you most grateful for today?*

....

....

....

DATE .... **YEAR** ....

FOOD: *What did you eat today?*

BREAKFAST: ....

Snack: ....

LUNCH: ....

Snack: ....

DINNER: ....

Snack: ....

DRINK: *What did you drink today?*

Any caffeinated drinks: ....

Any alcoholic drinks: ....

Any other drinks: ....

Any other drugs ingested: (including prescription, recreational, over the counter and nicotine) ....

....

QUICK CHECKLIST

WATER - how many litres? ▫   MEDITATION - how many minutes? ▫

SLEEP - how many hours? ▫   EXERCISE - how many minutes? ▫

LIFE EVENTS: *What happened today?*

....

....

....

EMOTIONS/THOUGHTS: *How did you feel today?*

....

....

....

CONCERNS LIST: *What bothered you most today?*

....

....

....

GRATITUDE LIST: *What are you most grateful for today?*

....

....

....

DATE .... **YEAR** ....

FOOD: *What did you eat today?*

BREAKFAST: ....

Snack: ....

LUNCH: ....

Snack: ....

DINNER: ....

Snack: ....

DRINK: *What did you drink today?*

Any caffeinated drinks: ....

Any alcoholic drinks: ....

Any other drinks: ....

Any other drugs ingested: (including prescription, recreational, over the counter and nicotine) ....

....

QUICK CHECKLIST

WATER - how many litres? ▢   MEDITATION - how many minutes? ▢

SLEEP - how many hours? ▢   EXERCISE - how many minutes? ▢

LIFE EVENTS: *What happened today?*

....

....

....

EMOTIONS/THOUGHTS: *How did you feel today?*

....

....

....

CONCERNS LIST: *What bothered you most today?*

....

....

....

GRATITUDE LIST: *What are you most grateful for today?*

....

....

....

DATE .... **YEAR** ....

FOOD: *What did you eat today?*

BREAKFAST: ....

Snack: ....

LUNCH: ....

Snack: ....

DINNER: ....

Snack: ....

DRINK: *What did you drink today?*

Any caffeinated drinks: ....

Any alcoholic drinks: ....

Any other drinks: ....

Any other drugs ingested: (including prescription, recreational, over the counter and nicotine) ....

....

QUICK CHECKLIST

WATER - how many litres? ▢   MEDITATION - how many minutes? ▢

SLEEP - how many hours? ▢   EXERCISE - how many minutes? ▢

LIFE EVENTS: *What happened today?*

....

....

....

EMOTIONS/THOUGHTS: *How did you feel today?*

....

....

....

CONCERNS LIST: *What bothered you most today?*

....

....

....

GRATITUDE LIST: *What are you most grateful for today?*

....

....

....

DATE .... **YEAR** ....

FOOD: *What did you eat today?*

BREAKFAST: ....

Snack: ....

LUNCH: ....

Snack: ....

DINNER: ....

Snack: ....

DRINK: *What did you drink today?*

Any caffeinated drinks: ....

Any alcoholic drinks: ....

Any other drinks: ....

Any other drugs ingested: (including prescription, recreational, over the counter and nicotine) ....

....

QUICK CHECKLIST

WATER - how many litres? ☐   MEDITATION - how many minutes? ☐

SLEEP - how many hours? ☐   EXERCISE - how many minutes? ☐

LIFE EVENTS: *What happened today?*

....

....

....

EMOTIONS/THOUGHTS: *How did you feel today?*

....

....

....

CONCERNS LIST: *What bothered you most today?*

....

....

....

GRATITUDE LIST: *What are you most grateful for today?*

....

....

....

DATE .... **YEAR** ....

FOOD: *What did you eat today?*

BREAKFAST: ....

Snack: ....

LUNCH: ....

Snack: ....

DINNER: ....

Snack: ....

DRINK: *What did you drink today?*

Any caffeinated drinks: ....

Any alcoholic drinks: ....

Any other drinks: ....

Any other drugs ingested: (including prescription, recreational, over the counter and nicotine) ....

....

QUICK CHECKLIST

WATER - how many litres? ☐   MEDITATION - how many minutes? ☐

SLEEP - how many hours? ☐   EXERCISE - how many minutes? ☐

LIFE EVENTS: *What happened today?*

....

....

....

EMOTIONS/THOUGHTS: *How did you feel today?*

....

....

....

CONCERNS LIST: *What bothered you most today?*

....

....

....

GRATITUDE LIST: *What are you most grateful for today?*

....

....

....

MONTH

SIX

anxiety

Everyone feels anxious sometimes. It's a normal response to stressful situations. For some people though, anxiety *becomes* the stressful problem, rather than it being the side-effect of a stressful problem. When you suffer with high anxiety, it can impair your life to a debilitating degree. It can be such a hard pattern to break. The happy news is, that it is absolutely possible to break free of it.

When anxiety occurs, your brain triggers a release of stress hormones such as cortisol and adrenaline. The surge of these powerful hormones causes physical reactions that are hard to ignore: your heart speeds up, you might get palpitations, your breathing pattern changes, you might feel weak, light-headed and shaky. Your temperature rises. Your throat feels dry and your palms feel clammy. Your muscles tense up and you're suddenly preoccupied by this uncomfortable heightened state of awareness.

There are so many symptoms of anxiety and the severity and combination will vary from person to person. Anxiety symptoms can be experienced constantly at low-level: maybe you're going through an on-going and challenging situation at work. Or they can strike suddenly; imagine that you're happily strolling down the street when a dog jumps over a fence and starts attacking you. The speed and intensity at which your body is being flooded by stress hormones will affect how you react to them.

This automatic process is amazing and hugely beneficial in certain situations. If you *were* to be attacked by a stroppy dog, the sudden influx of adrenaline would help you to either defend yourself (the fight response) or escape to safety (the flight response). These reactions enable us to act fast, think quick and prioritise whatever the immediate situation warrants. Unfortunately, this same process can go awry and get triggered when it's *not* needed or wanted. We might be sitting on the sofa trying to enjoy a nice cup of tea with a friend when suddenly we're in the grips of a panic attack. The symptoms that anxiety causes can be incredibly unsettling, especially when they seem to keep happening to an overwhelming degree in response to the slightest stressors. A trip to the shop for some people can prompt intense nervousness. Any social interaction can become an unbearable ordeal. The anticipatory fear of anxiety creates a pathological cycle that can then lead to all manner of additional problems: co-dependent relationships, binge-drinking, alcohol-dependence, reliance on prescription medication and other forms of substance abuse, depression, hypochondria and isolation.

As with most health problems, if you address the root cause of the problem, the symptoms of the problem will usually dissipate by themselves over time. So go back to all the healthy basics. Get journaling. Track your progress. Commit to helping yourself every single day. Make getting back on track your number one priority.

Strip away all of the unhealthy coping strategies that you might have incorporated into your life in order to distract, disguise or desensitise. Excessive alcohol use, or using any other drugs, to cope with uncomfortable symptoms will only mask the problem and potentially aggravate it even further. You might be successfully numbing out, but you're failing to address the root cause.

Embrace all of the good wholesome stuff. Learn about nutrition. Cook from scratch. Take up exercise. Dance. Read. Sing. Make sure you're getting enough sleep. Drink water. Invest in your friendships. Practice being more gentle with yourself where needed and be more firm with yourself when you need to be too. 'Treating yourself' to chocolate, cake and crisps every single day is categorically harmful to your health. Instead, learn to treat yourself with respect by choosing healthy alternatives: a cosy cat-nap, a green juice, a gym session or a bubble bath. Learn to truly appreciate and respect your health. Learn to enjoy nutritious food. Educate yourself about the effects of processed food and too much sugar. Be truly accountable for your own health and happiness. Responsibly research your symptoms. Join support groups. Talk to like-minded people. Gather tips and advice and try the ones that attract you.

Try your very best to untangle the underlying issues that create your surface symptoms and you'll stand a fantastic chance of feeling far happier and healthier in the long run.

MONTH .... YEAR ....

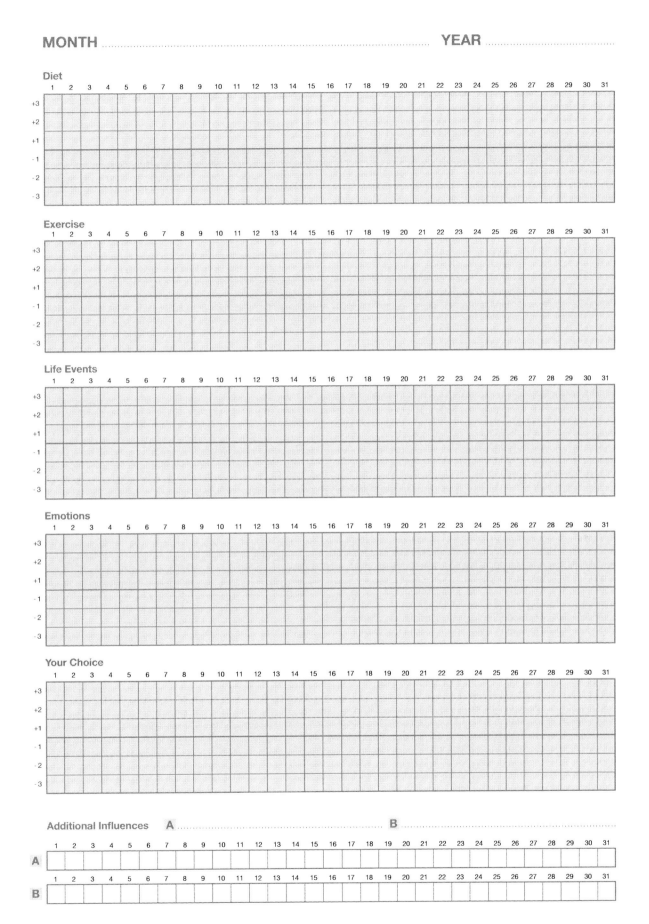

Diet

Exercise

Life Events

Emotions

Your Choice

Additional Influences   A ....   B ....

DATE .... **YEAR** ....

FOOD: *What did you eat today?*

BREAKFAST: ....

Snack: ....

LUNCH: ....

Snack: ....

DINNER: ....

Snack: ....

DRINK: *What did you drink today?*

Any caffeinated drinks: ....

Any alcoholic drinks: ....

Any other drinks: ....

Any other drugs ingested: (including prescription, recreational, over the counter and nicotine) ....

....

QUICK CHECKLIST

WATER - how many litres? ▢   MEDITATION - how many minutes? ▢

SLEEP - how many hours? ▢   EXERCISE - how many minutes? ▢

LIFE EVENTS: *What happened today?*

....

....

....

EMOTIONS/THOUGHTS: *How did you feel today?*

....

....

....

CONCERNS LIST: *What bothered you most today?*

....

....

....

GRATITUDE LIST: *What are you most grateful for today?*

....

....

....

DATE .... **YEAR** ....

FOOD: *What did you eat today?*

BREAKFAST: ....

Snack: ....

LUNCH: ....

Snack: ....

DINNER: ....

Snack: ....

DRINK: *What did you drink today?*

Any caffeinated drinks: ....

Any alcoholic drinks: ....

Any other drinks: ....

Any other drugs ingested: (including prescription, recreational, over the counter and nicotine) ....

....

QUICK CHECKLIST

WATER - how many litres? ▨   MEDITATION - how many minutes? ▨

SLEEP - how many hours? ▨   EXERCISE - how many minutes? ▨

LIFE EVENTS: *What happened today?*

....

....

....

EMOTIONS/THOUGHTS: *How did you feel today?*

....

....

....

CONCERNS LIST: *What bothered you most today?*

....

....

....

GRATITUDE LIST: *What are you most grateful for today?*

....

....

....

DATE .... **YEAR** ....

FOOD: *What did you eat today?*

BREAKFAST: ....

Snack: ....

LUNCH: ....

Snack: ....

DINNER: ....

Snack: ....

DRINK: *What did you drink today?*

Any caffeinated drinks: ....

Any alcoholic drinks: ....

Any other drinks: ....

Any other drugs ingested: (including prescription, recreational, over the counter and nicotine) ....

....

QUICK CHECKLIST

WATER - how many litres? ⬚   MEDITATION - how many minutes? ⬚

SLEEP - how many hours? ⬚   EXERCISE - how many minutes? ⬚

LIFE EVENTS: *What happened today?*

....

....

....

EMOTIONS/THOUGHTS: *How did you feel today?*

....

....

....

CONCERNS LIST: *What bothered you most today?*

....

....

....

GRATITUDE LIST: *What are you most grateful for today?*

....

....

....

DATE .... **YEAR** ....

FOOD: *What did you eat today?*

BREAKFAST: ....

Snack: ....

LUNCH: ....

Snack: ....

DINNER: ....

Snack: ....

DRINK: *What did you drink today?*

Any caffeinated drinks: ....

Any alcoholic drinks: ....

Any other drinks: ....

Any other drugs ingested: (including prescription, recreational, over the counter and nicotine) ....

....

QUICK CHECKLIST

WATER - how many litres? ▓   MEDITATION - how many minutes? ▓

SLEEP - how many hours? ▓   EXERCISE - how many minutes? ▓

LIFE EVENTS: *What happened today?*

....

....

....

EMOTIONS/THOUGHTS: *How did you feel today?*

....

....

....

CONCERNS LIST: *What bothered you most today?*

....

....

....

GRATITUDE LIST: *What are you most grateful for today?*

....

....

....

DATE .... YEAR ....

FOOD: *What did you eat today?*

BREAKFAST: ....

Snack: ....

LUNCH: ....

Snack: ....

DINNER: ....

Snack: ....

DRINK: *What did you drink today?*

Any caffeinated drinks: ....

Any alcoholic drinks: ....

Any other drinks: ....

Any other drugs ingested: (including prescription, recreational, over the counter and nicotine) ....

....

QUICK CHECKLIST

WATER - how many litres? ☐   MEDITATION - how many minutes? ☐

SLEEP - how many hours? ☐   EXERCISE - how many minutes? ☐

LIFE EVENTS: *What happened today?*

....

....

....

EMOTIONS/THOUGHTS: *How did you feel today?*

....

....

....

CONCERNS LIST: *What bothered you most today?*

....

....

....

GRATITUDE LIST: *What are you most grateful for today?*

....

....

....

DATE .... **YEAR** ....

FOOD: *What did you eat today?*

BREAKFAST: ....

Snack: ....

LUNCH: ....

Snack: ....

DINNER: ....

Snack: ....

DRINK: *What did you drink today?*

Any caffeinated drinks: ....

Any alcoholic drinks: ....

Any other drinks: ....

Any other drugs ingested: (including prescription, recreational, over the counter and nicotine) ....

....

QUICK CHECKLIST

WATER - how many litres? ▦   MEDITATION - how many minutes? ▦

SLEEP - how many hours? ▦   EXERCISE - how many minutes? ▦

LIFE EVENTS: *What happened today?*

....

....

....

EMOTIONS/THOUGHTS: *How did you feel today?*

....

....

....

CONCERNS LIST: *What bothered you most today?*

....

....

....

GRATITUDE LIST: *What are you most grateful for today?*

....

....

....

DATE .... **YEAR** ....

FOOD: *What did you eat today?*

BREAKFAST: ....

Snack: ....

LUNCH: ....

Snack: ....

DINNER: ....

Snack: ....

DRINK: *What did you drink today?*

Any caffeinated drinks: ....

Any alcoholic drinks: ....

Any other drinks: ....

Any other drugs ingested: (including prescription, recreational, over the counter and nicotine) ....

....

QUICK CHECKLIST

WATER - how many litres? ▢   MEDITATION - how many minutes? ▢

SLEEP - how many hours? ▢   EXERCISE - how many minutes? ▢

LIFE EVENTS: *What happened today?*

....

....

....

EMOTIONS/THOUGHTS: *How did you feel today?*

....

....

....

CONCERNS LIST: *What bothered you most today?*

....

....

....

GRATITUDE LIST: *What are you most grateful for today?*

....

....

....

DATE .... **YEAR** ....

FOOD: *What did you eat today?*

BREAKFAST: ....

Snack: ....

LUNCH: ....

Snack: ....

DINNER: ....

Snack: ....

DRINK: *What did you drink today?*

Any caffeinated drinks: ....

Any alcoholic drinks: ....

Any other drinks: ....

Any other drugs ingested: (including prescription, recreational, over the counter and nicotine) ....

....

QUICK CHECKLIST

WATER - how many litres? ☐   MEDITATION - how many minutes? ☐

SLEEP - how many hours? ☐   EXERCISE - how many minutes? ☐

LIFE EVENTS: *What happened today?*

....

....

....

EMOTIONS/THOUGHTS: *How did you feel today?*

....

....

....

CONCERNS LIST: *What bothered you most today?*

....

....

....

GRATITUDE LIST: *What are you most grateful for today?*

....

....

....

DATE .... YEAR ....

FOOD: *What did you eat today?*

BREAKFAST: ....

Snack: ....

LUNCH: ....

Snack: ....

DINNER: ....

Snack: ....

DRINK: *What did you drink today?*

Any caffeinated drinks: ....

Any alcoholic drinks: ....

Any other drinks: ....

Any other drugs ingested: (including prescription, recreational, over the counter and nicotine) ....

....

QUICK CHECKLIST

WATER - how many litres? ▢   MEDITATION - how many minutes? ▢

SLEEP - how many hours? ▢   EXERCISE - how many minutes? ▢

LIFE EVENTS: *What happened today?*

....

....

....

EMOTIONS/THOUGHTS: *How did you feel today?*

....

....

....

CONCERNS LIST: *What bothered you most today?*

....

....

....

GRATITUDE LIST: *What are you most grateful for today?*

....

....

....

DATE .... **YEAR** ....

FOOD: *What did you eat today?*

BREAKFAST: ....

Snack: ....

LUNCH: ....

Snack: ....

DINNER: ....

Snack: ....

DRINK: *What did you drink today?*

Any caffeinated drinks: ....

Any alcoholic drinks: ....

Any other drinks: ....

Any other drugs ingested: (including prescription, recreational, over the counter and nicotine) ....

....

QUICK CHECKLIST

WATER - how many litres? ▢   MEDITATION - how many minutes? ▢

SLEEP - how many hours? ▢   EXERCISE - how many minutes? ▢

LIFE EVENTS: *What happened today?*

....

....

....

EMOTIONS/THOUGHTS: *How did you feel today?*

....

....

....

CONCERNS LIST: *What bothered you most today?*

....

....

....

GRATITUDE LIST: *What are you most grateful for today?*

....

....

....

DATE .... YEAR ....

FOOD: *What did you eat today?*

BREAKFAST: ....

Snack: ....

LUNCH: ....

Snack: ....

DINNER: ....

Snack: ....

DRINK: *What did you drink today?*

Any caffeinated drinks: ....

Any alcoholic drinks: ....

Any other drinks: ....

Any other drugs ingested: (including prescription, recreational, over the counter and nicotine) ....

....

QUICK CHECKLIST

WATER - how many litres? ▨   MEDITATION - how many minutes? ▨

SLEEP - how many hours? ▨   EXERCISE - how many minutes? ▨

LIFE EVENTS: *What happened today?*

....

....

....

EMOTIONS/THOUGHTS: *How did you feel today?*

....

....

....

CONCERNS LIST: *What bothered you most today?*

....

....

....

GRATITUDE LIST: *What are you most grateful for today?*

....

....

....

DATE .... **YEAR** ....

FOOD: *What did you eat today?*

BREAKFAST: ....

Snack: ....

LUNCH: ....

Snack: ....

DINNER: ....

Snack: ....

DRINK: *What did you drink today?*

Any caffeinated drinks: ....

Any alcoholic drinks: ....

Any other drinks: ....

Any other drugs ingested: (including prescription, recreational, over the counter and nicotine) ....

....

QUICK CHECKLIST

WATER - how many litres? ▦   MEDITATION - how many minutes? ▦

SLEEP - how many hours? ▦   EXERCISE - how many minutes? ▦

LIFE EVENTS: *What happened today?*

....

....

....

EMOTIONS/THOUGHTS: *How did you feel today?*

....

....

....

CONCERNS LIST: *What bothered you most today?*

....

....

....

GRATITUDE LIST: *What are you most grateful for today?*

....

....

....

DATE .... **YEAR** ....

FOOD: *What did you eat today?*

BREAKFAST: ....

Snack: ....

LUNCH: ....

Snack: ....

DINNER: ....

Snack: ....

DRINK: *What did you drink today?*

Any caffeinated drinks: ....

Any alcoholic drinks: ....

Any other drinks: ....

Any other drugs ingested: (including prescription, recreational, over the counter and nicotine) ....

....

QUICK CHECKLIST

WATER - how many litres? ▓   MEDITATION - how many minutes? ▓

SLEEP - how many hours? ▓   EXERCISE - how many minutes? ▓

LIFE EVENTS: *What happened today?*

....

....

....

EMOTIONS/THOUGHTS: *How did you feel today?*

....

....

....

CONCERNS LIST: *What bothered you most today?*

....

....

....

GRATITUDE LIST: *What are you most grateful for today?*

....

....

....

DATE .... **YEAR** ....

FOOD: *What did you eat today?*

BREAKFAST: ....

Snack: ....

LUNCH: ....

Snack: ....

DINNER: ....

Snack: ....

DRINK: *What did you drink today?*

Any caffeinated drinks: ....

Any alcoholic drinks: ....

Any other drinks: ....

Any other drugs ingested: (including prescription, recreational, over the counter and nicotine) ....

....

QUICK CHECKLIST

WATER - how many litres? ⬜   MEDITATION - how many minutes? ⬜

SLEEP - how many hours? ⬜   EXERCISE - how many minutes? ⬜

LIFE EVENTS: *What happened today?*

....

....

....

EMOTIONS/THOUGHTS: *How did you feel today?*

....

....

....

CONCERNS LIST: *What bothered you most today?*

....

....

....

GRATITUDE LIST: *What are you most grateful for today?*

....

....

....

DATE .... YEAR ....

FOOD: *What did you eat today?*

BREAKFAST: ....

Snack: ....

LUNCH: ....

Snack: ....

DINNER: ....

Snack: ....

DRINK: *What did you drink today?*

Any caffeinated drinks: ....

Any alcoholic drinks: ....

Any other drinks: ....

Any other drugs ingested: (including prescription, recreational, over the counter and nicotine) ....

....

QUICK CHECKLIST

WATER - how many litres? ☐   MEDITATION - how many minutes? ☐

SLEEP - how many hours? ☐   EXERCISE - how many minutes? ☐

LIFE EVENTS: *What happened today?*

....

....

....

EMOTIONS/THOUGHTS: *How did you feel today?*

....

....

....

CONCERNS LIST: *What bothered you most today?*

....

....

....

GRATITUDE LIST: *What are you most grateful for today?*

....

....

....

DATE .... **YEAR** ....

FOOD: *What did you eat today?*

BREAKFAST: ....

Snack: ....

LUNCH: ....

Snack: ....

DINNER: ....

Snack: ....

DRINK: *What did you drink today?*

Any caffeinated drinks: ....

Any alcoholic drinks: ....

Any other drinks: ....

Any other drugs ingested: (including prescription, recreational, over the counter and nicotine) ....
....

QUICK CHECKLIST

WATER - how many litres? ▢   MEDITATION - how many minutes? ▢

SLEEP - how many hours? ▢   EXERCISE - how many minutes? ▢

LIFE EVENTS: *What happened today?*

....

....

....

EMOTIONS/THOUGHTS: *How did you feel today?*

....

....

....

CONCERNS LIST: *What bothered you most today?*

....

....

....

GRATITUDE LIST: *What are you most grateful for today?*

....

....

....

DATE .... **YEAR** ....

FOOD: *What did you eat today?*

BREAKFAST: ....

Snack: ....

LUNCH: ....

Snack: ....

DINNER: ....

Snack: ....

DRINK: *What did you drink today?*

Any caffeinated drinks: ....

Any alcoholic drinks: ....

Any other drinks: ....

Any other drugs ingested: (including prescription, recreational, over the counter and nicotine) ....

....

QUICK CHECKLIST

WATER - how many litres? ☐   MEDITATION - how many minutes? ☐

SLEEP - how many hours? ☐   EXERCISE - how many minutes? ☐

LIFE EVENTS: *What happened today?*

....

....

....

EMOTIONS/THOUGHTS: *How did you feel today?*

....

....

....

CONCERNS LIST: *What bothered you most today?*

....

....

....

GRATITUDE LIST: *What are you most grateful for today?*

....

....

....

DATE .... **YEAR** ....

FOOD: *What did you eat today?*

BREAKFAST: ....

Snack: ....

LUNCH: ....

Snack: ....

DINNER: ....

Snack: ....

DRINK: *What did you drink today?*

Any caffeinated drinks: ....

Any alcoholic drinks: ....

Any other drinks: ....

Any other drugs ingested: (including prescription, recreational, over the counter and nicotine) ....
....

QUICK CHECKLIST

WATER - how many litres? ☐   MEDITATION - how many minutes? ☐

SLEEP - how many hours? ☐   EXERCISE - how many minutes? ☐

LIFE EVENTS: *What happened today?*

....

....

....

EMOTIONS/THOUGHTS: *How did you feel today?*

....

....

....

CONCERNS LIST: *What bothered you most today?*

....

....

....

GRATITUDE LIST: *What are you most grateful for today?*

....

....

....

DATE .... **YEAR** ....

FOOD: *What did you eat today?*

BREAKFAST: ....

Snack: ....

LUNCH: ....

Snack: ....

DINNER: ....

Snack: ....

DRINK: *What did you drink today?*

Any caffeinated drinks: ....

Any alcoholic drinks: ....

Any other drinks: ....

Any other drugs ingested: (including prescription, recreational, over the counter and nicotine) ....

....

QUICK CHECKLIST

WATER - how many litres? ☐   MEDITATION - how many minutes? ☐

SLEEP - how many hours? ☐   EXERCISE - how many minutes? ☐

LIFE EVENTS: *What happened today?*

....

....

....

EMOTIONS/THOUGHTS: *How did you feel today?*

....

....

....

CONCERNS LIST: *What bothered you most today?*

....

....

....

GRATITUDE LIST: *What are you most grateful for today?*

....

....

....

DATE .... **YEAR** ....

FOOD: *What did you eat today?*

BREAKFAST: ....

Snack: ....

LUNCH: ....

Snack: ....

DINNER: ....

Snack: ....

DRINK: *What did you drink today?*

Any caffeinated drinks: ....

Any alcoholic drinks: ....

Any other drinks: ....

Any other drugs ingested: (including prescription, recreational, over the counter and nicotine) ....

....

QUICK CHECKLIST

WATER - how many litres? ☐   MEDITATION - how many minutes? ☐

SLEEP - how many hours? ☐   EXERCISE - how many minutes? ☐

LIFE EVENTS: *What happened today?*

....

....

....

EMOTIONS/THOUGHTS: *How did you feel today?*

....

....

....

CONCERNS LIST: *What bothered you most today?*

....

....

....

GRATITUDE LIST: *What are you most grateful for today?*

....

....

....

DATE .... **YEAR** ....

FOOD: *What did you eat today?*

BREAKFAST: ....

Snack: ....

LUNCH: ....

Snack: ....

DINNER: ....

Snack: ....

DRINK: *What did you drink today?*

Any caffeinated drinks: ....

Any alcoholic drinks: ....

Any other drinks: ....

Any other drugs ingested: (including prescription, recreational, over the counter and nicotine) ....

....

QUICK CHECKLIST

WATER - how many litres?   ▢   MEDITATION - how many minutes?   ▢

SLEEP - how many hours?   ▢   EXERCISE - how many minutes?   ▢

LIFE EVENTS: *What happened today?*

....

....

....

EMOTIONS/THOUGHTS: *How did you feel today?*

....

....

....

CONCERNS LIST: *What bothered you most today?*

....

....

....

GRATITUDE LIST: *What are you most grateful for today?*

....

....

....

DATE .... **YEAR** ....

FOOD: *What did you eat today?*

BREAKFAST: ....

Snack: ....

LUNCH: ....

Snack: ....

DINNER: ....

Snack: ....

DRINK: *What did you drink today?*

Any caffeinated drinks: ....

Any alcoholic drinks: ....

Any other drinks: ....

Any other drugs ingested: (including prescription, recreational, over the counter and nicotine) ....

....

QUICK CHECKLIST

WATER - how many litres? ▢   MEDITATION - how many minutes? ▢

SLEEP - how many hours? ▢   EXERCISE - how many minutes? ▢

LIFE EVENTS: *What happened today?*

....

....

....

EMOTIONS/THOUGHTS: *How did you feel today?*

....

....

....

CONCERNS LIST: *What bothered you most today?*

....

....

....

GRATITUDE LIST: *What are you most grateful for today?*

....

....

....

DATE .... **YEAR** ....

FOOD: *What did you eat today?*

BREAKFAST: ....

Snack: ....

LUNCH: ....

Snack: ....

DINNER: ....

Snack: ....

DRINK: *What did you drink today?*

Any caffeinated drinks: ....

Any alcoholic drinks: ....

Any other drinks: ....

Any other drugs ingested: (including prescription, recreational, over the counter and nicotine) ....

....

QUICK CHECKLIST

WATER - how many litres? ☐   MEDITATION - how many minutes? ☐

SLEEP - how many hours? ☐   EXERCISE - how many minutes? ☐

LIFE EVENTS: *What happened today?*

....

....

....

EMOTIONS/THOUGHTS: *How did you feel today?*

....

....

....

CONCERNS LIST: *What bothered you most today?*

....

....

....

GRATITUDE LIST: *What are you most grateful for today?*

....

....

....

DATE .... **YEAR** ....

FOOD: *What did you eat today?*

BREAKFAST: ....

Snack: ....

LUNCH: ....

Snack: ....

DINNER: ....

Snack: ....

DRINK: *What did you drink today?*

Any caffeinated drinks: ....

Any alcoholic drinks: ....

Any other drinks: ....

Any other drugs ingested: (including prescription, recreational, over the counter and nicotine) ....

....

QUICK CHECKLIST

WATER - how many litres? ▨   MEDITATION - how many minutes? ▨

SLEEP - how many hours? ▨   EXERCISE - how many minutes? ▨

LIFE EVENTS: *What happened today?*

....

....

....

EMOTIONS/THOUGHTS: *How did you feel today?*

....

....

....

CONCERNS LIST: *What bothered you most today?*

....

....

....

GRATITUDE LIST: *What are you most grateful for today?*

....

....

....

DATE .... **YEAR** ....

FOOD: *What did you eat today?*

BREAKFAST: ....

Snack: ....

LUNCH: ....

Snack: ....

DINNER: ....

Snack: ....

DRINK: *What did you drink today?*

Any caffeinated drinks: ....

Any alcoholic drinks: ....

Any other drinks: ....

Any other drugs ingested: (including prescription, recreational, over the counter and nicotine) ....

....

QUICK CHECKLIST

WATER - how many litres? ▢   MEDITATION - how many minutes? ▢

SLEEP - how many hours? ▢   EXERCISE - how many minutes? ▢

LIFE EVENTS: *What happened today?*

....

....

....

EMOTIONS/THOUGHTS: *How did you feel today?*

....

....

....

CONCERNS LIST: *What bothered you most today?*

....

....

....

GRATITUDE LIST: *What are you most grateful for today?*

....

....

....

DATE .... **YEAR** ....

FOOD: *What did you eat today?*

BREAKFAST: ....

Snack: ....

LUNCH: ....

Snack: ....

DINNER: ....

Snack: ....

DRINK: *What did you drink today?*

Any caffeinated drinks: ....

Any alcoholic drinks: ....

Any other drinks: ....

Any other drugs ingested: (including prescription, recreational, over the counter and nicotine) ....

....

QUICK CHECKLIST

WATER - how many litres? ▨   MEDITATION - how many minutes? ▨

SLEEP - how many hours? ▨   EXERCISE - how many minutes? ▨

LIFE EVENTS: *What happened today?*

....

....

....

EMOTIONS/THOUGHTS: *How did you feel today?*

....

....

....

CONCERNS LIST: *What bothered you most today?*

....

....

....

GRATITUDE LIST: *What are you most grateful for today?*

....

....

....

DATE .... **YEAR** ....

FOOD: *What did you eat today?*

BREAKFAST: ....

Snack: ....

LUNCH: ....

Snack: ....

DINNER: ....

Snack: ....

DRINK: *What did you drink today?*

Any caffeinated drinks: ....

Any alcoholic drinks: ....

Any other drinks: ....

Any other drugs ingested: (including prescription, recreational, over the counter and nicotine) ....

....

QUICK CHECKLIST

WATER - how many litres? ☐   MEDITATION - how many minutes? ☐

SLEEP - how many hours? ☐   EXERCISE - how many minutes? ☐

LIFE EVENTS: *What happened today?*

....

....

....

EMOTIONS/THOUGHTS: *How did you feel today?*

....

....

....

CONCERNS LIST: *What bothered you most today?*

....

....

....

GRATITUDE LIST: *What are you most grateful for today?*

....

....

....

DATE .... **YEAR** ....

FOOD: *What did you eat today?*

BREAKFAST: ....

Snack: ....

LUNCH: ....

Snack: ....

DINNER: ....

Snack: ....

DRINK: *What did you drink today?*

Any caffeinated drinks: ....

Any alcoholic drinks: ....

Any other drinks: ....

Any other drugs ingested: (including prescription, recreational, over the counter and nicotine) ....

....

QUICK CHECKLIST

WATER - how many litres? ▢   MEDITATION - how many minutes? ▢

SLEEP - how many hours? ▢   EXERCISE - how many minutes? ▢

LIFE EVENTS: *What happened today?*

....

....

....

EMOTIONS/THOUGHTS: *How did you feel today?*

....

....

....

CONCERNS LIST: *What bothered you most today?*

....

....

....

GRATITUDE LIST: *What are you most grateful for today?*

....

....

....

DATE .... **YEAR** ....

FOOD: *What did you eat today?*

BREAKFAST: ....

Snack: ....

LUNCH: ....

Snack: ....

DINNER: ....

Snack: ....

DRINK: *What did you drink today?*

Any caffeinated drinks: ....

Any alcoholic drinks: ....

Any other drinks: ....

Any other drugs ingested: (including prescription, recreational, over the counter and nicotine) ....

....

QUICK CHECKLIST

WATER - how many litres? ☐   MEDITATION - how many minutes? ☐

SLEEP - how many hours? ☐   EXERCISE - how many minutes? ☐

LIFE EVENTS: *What happened today?*

....

....

....

EMOTIONS/THOUGHTS: *How did you feel today?*

....

....

....

CONCERNS LIST: *What bothered you most today?*

....

....

....

GRATITUDE LIST: *What are you most grateful for today?*

....

....

....

DATE .... **YEAR** ....

FOOD: *What did you eat today?*

BREAKFAST: ....

Snack: ....

LUNCH: ....

Snack: ....

DINNER: ....

Snack: ....

DRINK: *What did you drink today?*

Any caffeinated drinks: ....

Any alcoholic drinks: ....

Any other drinks: ....

Any other drugs ingested: (including prescription, recreational, over the counter and nicotine) ....

....

QUICK CHECKLIST

WATER - how many litres? ▨   MEDITATION - how many minutes? ▨

SLEEP - how many hours? ▨   EXERCISE - how many minutes? ▨

LIFE EVENTS: *What happened today?*

....

....

....

EMOTIONS/THOUGHTS: *How did you feel today?*

....

....

....

CONCERNS LIST: *What bothered you most today?*

....

....

....

GRATITUDE LIST: *What are you most grateful for today?*

....

....

....

DATE .... **YEAR** ....

FOOD: *What did you eat today?*

BREAKFAST: ....

Snack: ....

LUNCH: ....

Snack: ....

DINNER: ....

Snack: ....

DRINK: *What did you drink today?*

Any caffeinated drinks: ....

Any alcoholic drinks: ....

Any other drinks: ....

Any other drugs ingested: (including prescription, recreational, over the counter and nicotine) ....
....

QUICK CHECKLIST

WATER - how many litres? ▢   MEDITATION - how many minutes? ▢

SLEEP - how many hours? ▢   EXERCISE - how many minutes? ▢

LIFE EVENTS: *What happened today?*

....

....

....

EMOTIONS/THOUGHTS: *How did you feel today?*

....

....

....

CONCERNS LIST: *What bothered you most today?*

....

....

....

GRATITUDE LIST: *What are you most grateful for today?*

....

....

....

MONTH SEVEN

<u>addiction, compulsion and dependency</u>

Addiction is a spectrum condition that is characterised by the compulsive engagement in 'rewarding' stimuli despite the negative consequences. Most people are, or have been at some point, addicted to some thing, substance or behaviour - to some degree or another. It's easy to get tangled up in a downward spiral of denial and repetition and not even realise that you're struggling. Bad habits can become just another cyclical narrative of our lives, things we make allowances and excuses for. Things we're not too happy about but have come to depend on. Things that create or exacerbate more problems than they solve. Things that we're not completely honest with ourselves or others about. (Alcohol, for example, because it's a legally promoted and socially pushed drug, is super easy to develop an unhealthy relationship with.)

The issue of addiction is so multi-faceted and complex that it's under constant debate and study. Suffice it to say that if you feel controlled, compelled, stuck in a rut, unhappy or confused as to why you feel the recurrent need to engage in any behaviour or substance that routinely generates negative consequences, then that's a good enough reason to do something about it.

I believe that anything we do compulsively/destructively is just serving as a distraction from an underlying problem that we've yet to resolve. I think this goes for anybody who's tangled up in unhealthy habits with any substance or behaviour: alcohol, any other drug (legal or illegal, prescribed or otherwise), co-dependent relationships, sex, food, gambling, pornography, shopping etc. You'll get additional problems springing up that are directly related to those things the longer and harder you abuse them: illness, depression, anxiety, heartbreak, obesity, eating disorders, mounting debt etc, but the underlying drivers are often nothing to do with the surface problem. Addiction is pandemic. It's part of the human condition. It comes in many forms, to many things, to varying degrees. No two examples will be identical. In the same way that no two examples of people struggling with depression or anxiety will be identical. Each case will have as many similarities as differences. There is no one recovery method. This is why I created The Off The Rocks Journal in the first place - so that each individual could accurately and consistently assess their own lives, their own issues, their own triggers and track their own progress. So that they could take better control of their own problem areas and their own health and their own happiness.

Ultimately, it doesn't matter whether you believe you are hopelessly addicted or consciously choosing to repeatedly indulge in a bad habit. The negative outcome and the control that the thing (whatever it is), has over you, is the same, regardless of semantics and there is a happier, healthier way to live, I promise you.

MONTH .... **YEAR** ....

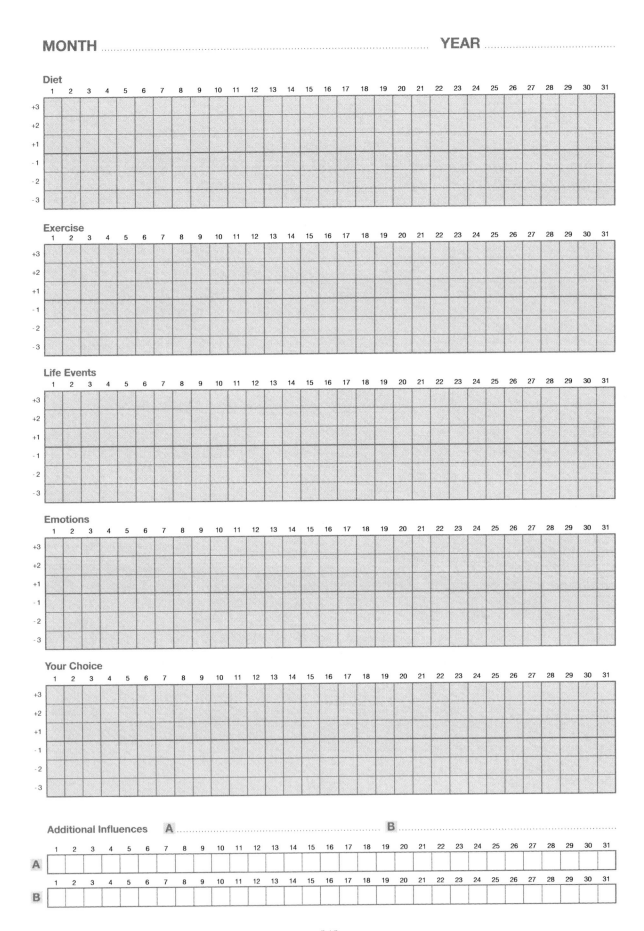

Diet

Exercise

Life Events

Emotions

Your Choice

Additional Influences   **A** ....   **B** ....

DATE .... **YEAR** ....

FOOD: *What did you eat today?*

BREAKFAST: ....

Snack: ....

LUNCH: ....

Snack: ....

DINNER: ....

Snack: ....

DRINK: *What did you drink today?*

Any caffeinated drinks: ....

Any alcoholic drinks: ....

Any other drinks: ....

Any other drugs ingested: (including prescription, recreational, over the counter and nicotine) ....

....

QUICK CHECKLIST

WATER - how many litres? ▨   MEDITATION - how many minutes? ▨

SLEEP - how many hours? ▨   EXERCISE - how many minutes? ▨

LIFE EVENTS: *What happened today?*

....

....

....

EMOTIONS/THOUGHTS: *How did you feel today?*

....

....

....

CONCERNS LIST: *What bothered you most today?*

....

....

....

GRATITUDE LIST: *What are you most grateful for today?*

....

....

....

DATE .... **YEAR** ....

FOOD: *What did you eat today?*

BREAKFAST: ....

Snack: ....

LUNCH: ....

Snack: ....

DINNER: ....

Snack: ....

DRINK: *What did you drink today?*

Any caffeinated drinks: ....

Any alcoholic drinks: ....

Any other drinks: ....

Any other drugs ingested: (including prescription, recreational, over the counter and nicotine) ....

....

QUICK CHECKLIST

WATER - how many litres? ☐   MEDITATION - how many minutes? ☐

SLEEP - how many hours? ☐   EXERCISE - how many minutes? ☐

LIFE EVENTS: *What happened today?*

....

....

....

EMOTIONS/THOUGHTS: *How did you feel today?*

....

....

....

CONCERNS LIST: *What bothered you most today?*

....

....

....

GRATITUDE LIST: *What are you most grateful for today?*

....

....

....

DATE .... **YEAR** ....

FOOD: *What did you eat today?*

BREAKFAST: ....

Snack: ....

LUNCH: ....

Snack: ....

DINNER: ....

Snack: ....

DRINK: *What did you drink today?*

Any caffeinated drinks: ....

Any alcoholic drinks: ....

Any other drinks: ....

Any other drugs ingested: (including prescription, recreational, over the counter and nicotine) ....

....

QUICK CHECKLIST

WATER - how many litres? ☐   MEDITATION - how many minutes? ☐

SLEEP - how many hours? ☐   EXERCISE - how many minutes? ☐

LIFE EVENTS: *What happened today?*

....

....

....

EMOTIONS/THOUGHTS: *How did you feel today?*

....

....

....

CONCERNS LIST: *What bothered you most today?*

....

....

....

GRATITUDE LIST: *What are you most grateful for today?*

....

....

....

DATE .... **YEAR** ....

FOOD: *What did you eat today?*

BREAKFAST: ....

Snack: ....

LUNCH: ....

Snack: ....

DINNER: ....

Snack: ....

DRINK: *What did you drink today?*

Any caffeinated drinks: ....

Any alcoholic drinks: ....

Any other drinks: ....

Any other drugs ingested: (including prescription, recreational, over the counter and nicotine) ....

....

QUICK CHECKLIST

WATER - how many litres? ▢   MEDITATION - how many minutes? ▢

SLEEP - how many hours? ▢   EXERCISE - how many minutes? ▢

LIFE EVENTS: *What happened today?*

....

....

....

EMOTIONS/THOUGHTS: *How did you feel today?*

....

....

....

CONCERNS LIST: *What bothered you most today?*

....

....

....

GRATITUDE LIST: *What are you most grateful for today?*

....

....

....

DATE .... **YEAR** ....

FOOD: *What did you eat today?*

BREAKFAST: ....

Snack: ....

LUNCH: ....

Snack: ....

DINNER: ....

Snack: ....

DRINK: *What did you drink today?*

Any caffeinated drinks: ....

Any alcoholic drinks: ....

Any other drinks: ....

Any other drugs ingested: (including prescription, recreational, over the counter and nicotine) ....

....

QUICK CHECKLIST

WATER - how many litres? ▨   MEDITATION - how many minutes? ▨

SLEEP - how many hours? ▨   EXERCISE - how many minutes? ▨

LIFE EVENTS: *What happened today?*

....

....

....

EMOTIONS/THOUGHTS: *How did you feel today?*

....

....

....

CONCERNS LIST: *What bothered you most today?*

....

....

....

GRATITUDE LIST: *What are you most grateful for today?*

....

....

....

DATE .... **YEAR** ....

FOOD: *What did you eat today?*

BREAKFAST: ....

Snack: ....

LUNCH: ....

Snack: ....

DINNER: ....

Snack: ....

DRINK: *What did you drink today?*

Any caffeinated drinks: ....

Any alcoholic drinks: ....

Any other drinks: ....

Any other drugs ingested: (including prescription, recreational, over the counter and nicotine) ....

....

QUICK CHECKLIST

WATER - how many litres? ☐   MEDITATION - how many minutes? ☐

SLEEP - how many hours? ☐   EXERCISE - how many minutes? ☐

LIFE EVENTS: *What happened today?*

....

....

....

EMOTIONS/THOUGHTS: *How did you feel today?*

....

....

....

CONCERNS LIST: *What bothered you most today?*

....

....

....

GRATITUDE LIST: *What are you most grateful for today?*

....

....

....

DATE .... **YEAR** ....

FOOD: *What did you eat today?*

BREAKFAST: ....

Snack: ....

LUNCH: ....

Snack: ....

DINNER: ....

Snack: ....

DRINK: *What did you drink today?*

Any caffeinated drinks: ....

Any alcoholic drinks: ....

Any other drinks: ....

Any other drugs ingested: (including prescription, recreational, over the counter and nicotine) ....

....

QUICK CHECKLIST

WATER - how many litres? ▨   MEDITATION - how many minutes? ▨

SLEEP - how many hours? ▨   EXERCISE - how many minutes? ▨

LIFE EVENTS: *What happened today?*

....

....

....

EMOTIONS/THOUGHTS: *How did you feel today?*

....

....

....

CONCERNS LIST: *What bothered you most today?*

....

....

....

GRATITUDE LIST: *What are you most grateful for today?*

....

....

....

DATE .... **YEAR** ....

FOOD: *What did you eat today?*

BREAKFAST: ....

Snack: ....

LUNCH: ....

Snack: ....

DINNER: ....

Snack: ....

DRINK: *What did you drink today?*

Any caffeinated drinks: ....

Any alcoholic drinks: ....

Any other drinks: ....

Any other drugs ingested: (including prescription, recreational, over the counter and nicotine) ....

....

QUICK CHECKLIST

WATER - how many litres? ▢   MEDITATION - how many minutes? ▢

SLEEP - how many hours? ▢   EXERCISE - how many minutes? ▢

LIFE EVENTS: *What happened today?*

....

....

....

EMOTIONS/THOUGHTS: *How did you feel today?*

....

....

....

CONCERNS LIST: *What bothered you most today?*

....

....

....

GRATITUDE LIST: *What are you most grateful for today?*

....

....

....

DATE .... **YEAR** ....

FOOD: *What did you eat today?*

BREAKFAST: ....

Snack: ....

LUNCH: ....

Snack: ....

DINNER: ....

Snack: ....

DRINK: *What did you drink today?*

Any caffeinated drinks: ....

Any alcoholic drinks: ....

Any other drinks: ....

Any other drugs ingested: (including prescription, recreational, over the counter and nicotine) ....

....

QUICK CHECKLIST

WATER - how many litres? ▧   MEDITATION - how many minutes? ▧

SLEEP - how many hours? ▧   EXERCISE - how many minutes? ▧

LIFE EVENTS: *What happened today?*

....

....

....

EMOTIONS/THOUGHTS: *How did you feel today?*

....

....

....

CONCERNS LIST: *What bothered you most today?*

....

....

....

GRATITUDE LIST: *What are you most grateful for today?*

....

....

....

DATE .... **YEAR** ....

FOOD: *What did you eat today?*

BREAKFAST: ....

Snack: ....

LUNCH: ....

Snack: ....

DINNER: ....

Snack: ....

DRINK: *What did you drink today?*

Any caffeinated drinks: ....

Any alcoholic drinks: ....

Any other drinks: ....

Any other drugs ingested: (including prescription, recreational, over the counter and nicotine) ....

....

QUICK CHECKLIST

WATER - how many litres? ☐   MEDITATION - how many minutes? ☐

SLEEP - how many hours? ☐   EXERCISE - how many minutes? ☐

LIFE EVENTS: *What happened today?*

....

....

....

EMOTIONS/THOUGHTS: *How did you feel today?*

....

....

....

CONCERNS LIST: *What bothered you most today?*

....

....

....

GRATITUDE LIST: *What are you most grateful for today?*

....

....

....

DATE .... **YEAR** ....

FOOD: *What did you eat today?*

BREAKFAST: ....

Snack: ....

LUNCH: ....

Snack: ....

DINNER: ....

Snack: ....

DRINK: *What did you drink today?*

Any caffeinated drinks: ....

Any alcoholic drinks: ....

Any other drinks: ....

Any other drugs ingested: (including prescription, recreational, over the counter and nicotine) ....

....

QUICK CHECKLIST

WATER - how many litres? ▓   MEDITATION - how many minutes? ▓

SLEEP - how many hours? ▓   EXERCISE - how many minutes? ▓

LIFE EVENTS: *What happened today?*

....

....

....

EMOTIONS/THOUGHTS: *How did you feel today?*

....

....

....

CONCERNS LIST: *What bothered you most today?*

....

....

....

GRATITUDE LIST: *What are you most grateful for today?*

....

....

....

DATE .... **YEAR** ....

FOOD: *What did you eat today?*

BREAKFAST: ....

Snack: ....

LUNCH: ....

Snack: ....

DINNER: ....

Snack: ....

DRINK: *What did you drink today?*

Any caffeinated drinks: ....

Any alcoholic drinks: ....

Any other drinks: ....

Any other drugs ingested: (including prescription, recreational, over the counter and nicotine) ....

....

QUICK CHECKLIST

WATER - how many litres? ▢   MEDITATION - how many minutes? ▢

SLEEP - how many hours? ▢   EXERCISE - how many minutes? ▢

LIFE EVENTS: *What happened today?*

....

....

....

EMOTIONS/THOUGHTS: *How did you feel today?*

....

....

....

CONCERNS LIST: *What bothered you most today?*

....

....

....

GRATITUDE LIST: *What are you most grateful for today?*

....

....

....

DATE .... **YEAR** ....

FOOD: *What did you eat today?*

BREAKFAST: ....

Snack: ....

LUNCH: ....

Snack: ....

DINNER: ....

Snack: ....

DRINK: *What did you drink today?*

Any caffeinated drinks: ....

Any alcoholic drinks: ....

Any other drinks: ....

Any other drugs ingested: (including prescription, recreational, over the counter and nicotine) ....

....

QUICK CHECKLIST

WATER - how many litres? ▨   MEDITATION - how many minutes? ▨

SLEEP - how many hours? ▨   EXERCISE - how many minutes? ▨

LIFE EVENTS: *What happened today?*

....

....

....

EMOTIONS/THOUGHTS: *How did you feel today?*

....

....

....

CONCERNS LIST: *What bothered you most today?*

....

....

....

GRATITUDE LIST: *What are you most grateful for today?*

....

....

....

DATE .... **YEAR** ....

FOOD: *What did you eat today?*

BREAKFAST: ....

Snack: ....

LUNCH: ....

Snack: ....

DINNER: ....

Snack: ....

DRINK: *What did you drink today?*

Any caffeinated drinks: ....

Any alcoholic drinks: ....

Any other drinks: ....

Any other drugs ingested: (including prescription, recreational, over the counter and nicotine) ....

....

QUICK CHECKLIST

WATER - how many litres? ▢   MEDITATION - how many minutes? ▢

SLEEP - how many hours? ▢   EXERCISE - how many minutes? ▢

LIFE EVENTS: *What happened today?*

....

....

....

EMOTIONS/THOUGHTS: *How did you feel today?*

....

....

....

CONCERNS LIST: *What bothered you most today?*

....

....

....

GRATITUDE LIST: *What are you most grateful for today?*

....

....

....

DATE .... **YEAR** ....

FOOD: *What did you eat today?*

BREAKFAST: ....

Snack: ....

LUNCH: ....

Snack: ....

DINNER: ....

Snack: ....

DRINK: *What did you drink today?*

Any caffeinated drinks: ....

Any alcoholic drinks: ....

Any other drinks: ....

Any other drugs ingested: (including prescription, recreational, over the counter and nicotine) ....

....

QUICK CHECKLIST

WATER - how many litres? ▨   MEDITATION - how many minutes? ▨

SLEEP - how many hours? ▨   EXERCISE - how many minutes? ▨

LIFE EVENTS: *What happened today?*

....

....

....

EMOTIONS/THOUGHTS: *How did you feel today?*

....

....

....

CONCERNS LIST: *What bothered you most today?*

....

....

....

GRATITUDE LIST: *What are you most grateful for today?*

....

....

....

DATE .... YEAR ....

FOOD: *What did you eat today?*

BREAKFAST: ....

Snack: ....

LUNCH: ....

Snack: ....

DINNER: ....

Snack: ....

DRINK: *What did you drink today?*

Any caffeinated drinks: ....

Any alcoholic drinks: ....

Any other drinks: ....

Any other drugs ingested: (including prescription, recreational, over the counter and nicotine) ....

....

QUICK CHECKLIST

WATER - how many litres? ☐   MEDITATION - how many minutes? ☐

SLEEP - how many hours? ☐   EXERCISE - how many minutes? ☐

LIFE EVENTS: *What happened today?*

....

....

....

EMOTIONS/THOUGHTS: *How did you feel today?*

....

....

....

CONCERNS LIST: *What bothered you most today?*

....

....

....

GRATITUDE LIST: *What are you most grateful for today?*

....

....

....

DATE .... **YEAR** ....

FOOD: *What did you eat today?*

BREAKFAST: ....

Snack: ....

LUNCH: ....

Snack: ....

DINNER: ....

Snack: ....

DRINK: *What did you drink today?*

Any caffeinated drinks: ....

Any alcoholic drinks: ....

Any other drinks: ....

Any other drugs ingested: (including prescription, recreational, over the counter and nicotine) ....

....

QUICK CHECKLIST

WATER - how many litres? ▨   MEDITATION - how many minutes? ▨

SLEEP - how many hours? ▨   EXERCISE - how many minutes? ▨

LIFE EVENTS: *What happened today?*

....

....

....

EMOTIONS/THOUGHTS: *How did you feel today?*

....

....

....

CONCERNS LIST: *What bothered you most today?*

....

....

....

GRATITUDE LIST: *What are you most grateful for today?*

....

....

....

DATE .... **YEAR** ....

FOOD: *What did you eat today?*

BREAKFAST: ....

Snack: ....

LUNCH: ....

Snack: ....

DINNER: ....

Snack: ....

DRINK: *What did you drink today?*

Any caffeinated drinks: ....

Any alcoholic drinks: ....

Any other drinks: ....

Any other drugs ingested: (including prescription, recreational, over the counter and nicotine) ....
....

QUICK CHECKLIST

WATER - how many litres? ☐   MEDITATION - how many minutes? ☐

SLEEP - how many hours? ☐   EXERCISE - how many minutes? ☐

LIFE EVENTS: *What happened today?*

....

....

....

EMOTIONS/THOUGHTS: *How did you feel today?*

....

....

....

CONCERNS LIST: *What bothered you most today?*

....

....

....

GRATITUDE LIST: *What are you most grateful for today?*

....

....

....

DATE .... **YEAR** ....

FOOD: *What did you eat today?*

BREAKFAST: ....

Snack: ....

LUNCH: ....

Snack: ....

DINNER: ....

Snack: ....

DRINK: *What did you drink today?*

Any caffeinated drinks: ....

Any alcoholic drinks: ....

Any other drinks: ....

Any other drugs ingested: (including prescription, recreational, over the counter and nicotine) ....

....

QUICK CHECKLIST

WATER - how many litres? ▢   MEDITATION - how many minutes? ▢

SLEEP - how many hours? ▢   EXERCISE - how many minutes? ▢

LIFE EVENTS: *What happened today?*

....

....

....

EMOTIONS/THOUGHTS: *How did you feel today?*

....

....

....

CONCERNS LIST: *What bothered you most today?*

....

....

....

GRATITUDE LIST: *What are you most grateful for today?*

....

....

....

DATE .... **YEAR** ....

FOOD: *What did you eat today?*

BREAKFAST: ....

Snack: ....

LUNCH: ....

Snack: ....

DINNER: ....

Snack: ....

DRINK: *What did you drink today?*

Any caffeinated drinks: ....

Any alcoholic drinks: ....

Any other drinks: ....

Any other drugs ingested: (including prescription, recreational, over the counter and nicotine) ....

....

QUICK CHECKLIST

WATER - how many litres? ☐   MEDITATION - how many minutes? ☐

SLEEP - how many hours? ☐   EXERCISE - how many minutes? ☐

LIFE EVENTS: *What happened today?*

....

....

....

EMOTIONS/THOUGHTS: *How did you feel today?*

....

....

....

CONCERNS LIST: *What bothered you most today?*

....

....

....

GRATITUDE LIST: *What are you most grateful for today?*

....

....

....

DATE .... **YEAR** ....

FOOD: *What did you eat today?*

BREAKFAST: ....

Snack: ....

LUNCH: ....

Snack: ....

DINNER: ....

Snack: ....

DRINK: *What did you drink today?*

Any caffeinated drinks: ....

Any alcoholic drinks: ....

Any other drinks: ....

Any other drugs ingested: (including prescription, recreational, over the counter and nicotine) ....

....

QUICK CHECKLIST

WATER - how many litres? ▢   MEDITATION - how many minutes? ▢

SLEEP - how many hours? ▢   EXERCISE - how many minutes? ▢

LIFE EVENTS: *What happened today?*

....

....

....

EMOTIONS/THOUGHTS: *How did you feel today?*

....

....

....

CONCERNS LIST: *What bothered you most today?*

....

....

....

GRATITUDE LIST: *What are you most grateful for today?*

....

....

....

DATE .... **YEAR** ....

FOOD: *What did you eat today?*

BREAKFAST: ....

Snack: ....

LUNCH: ....

Snack: ....

DINNER: ....

Snack: ....

DRINK: *What did you drink today?*

Any caffeinated drinks: ....

Any alcoholic drinks: ....

Any other drinks: ....

Any other drugs ingested: (including prescription, recreational, over the counter and nicotine) ....
....

QUICK CHECKLIST

WATER - how many litres?   ▢   MEDITATION - how many minutes?   ▢

SLEEP - how many hours?   ▢   EXERCISE - how many minutes?   ▢

LIFE EVENTS: *What happened today?*

....
....
....

EMOTIONS/THOUGHTS: *How did you feel today?*

....
....
....

CONCERNS LIST: *What bothered you most today?*

....
....
....

GRATITUDE LIST: *What are you most grateful for today?*

....
....
....

DATE .... **YEAR** ....

FOOD: *What did you eat today?*

BREAKFAST: ....

Snack: ....

LUNCH: ....

Snack: ....

DINNER: ....

Snack: ....

DRINK: *What did you drink today?*

Any caffeinated drinks: ....

Any alcoholic drinks: ....

Any other drinks: ....

Any other drugs ingested: (including prescription, recreational, over the counter and nicotine) ....

....

QUICK CHECKLIST

WATER - how many litres? ▢   MEDITATION - how many minutes? ▢

SLEEP - how many hours? ▢   EXERCISE - how many minutes? ▢

LIFE EVENTS: *What happened today?*

....

....

....

EMOTIONS/THOUGHTS: *How did you feel today?*

....

....

....

CONCERNS LIST: *What bothered you most today?*

....

....

....

GRATITUDE LIST: *What are you most grateful for today?*

....

....

....

DATE .... YEAR ....

FOOD: *What did you eat today?*

BREAKFAST: ....

Snack: ....

LUNCH: ....

Snack: ....

DINNER: ....

Snack: ....

DRINK: *What did you drink today?*

Any caffeinated drinks: ....

Any alcoholic drinks: ....

Any other drinks: ....

Any other drugs ingested: (including prescription, recreational, over the counter and nicotine) ....

....

QUICK CHECKLIST

WATER - how many litres? ☐   MEDITATION - how many minutes? ☐

SLEEP - how many hours? ☐   EXERCISE - how many minutes? ☐

LIFE EVENTS: *What happened today?*

....

....

....

EMOTIONS/THOUGHTS: *How did you feel today?*

....

....

....

CONCERNS LIST: *What bothered you most today?*

....

....

....

GRATITUDE LIST: *What are you most grateful for today?*

....

....

....

DATE .... **YEAR** ....

FOOD: *What did you eat today?*

BREAKFAST: ....

Snack: ....

LUNCH: ....

Snack: ....

DINNER: ....

Snack: ....

DRINK: *What did you drink today?*

Any caffeinated drinks: ....

Any alcoholic drinks: ....

Any other drinks: ....

Any other drugs ingested: (including prescription, recreational, over the counter and nicotine) ....

....

QUICK CHECKLIST

WATER - how many litres? ☐   MEDITATION - how many minutes? ☐

SLEEP - how many hours? ☐   EXERCISE - how many minutes? ☐

LIFE EVENTS: *What happened today?*

....

....

....

EMOTIONS/THOUGHTS: *How did you feel today?*

....

....

....

CONCERNS LIST: *What bothered you most today?*

....

....

....

GRATITUDE LIST: *What are you most grateful for today?*

....

....

....

DATE .... **YEAR** ....

FOOD: *What did you eat today?*

BREAKFAST: ....

Snack: ....

LUNCH: ....

Snack: ....

DINNER: ....

Snack: ....

DRINK: *What did you drink today?*

Any caffeinated drinks: ....

Any alcoholic drinks: ....

Any other drinks: ....

Any other drugs ingested: (including prescription, recreational, over the counter and nicotine) ....
....

QUICK CHECKLIST

WATER - how many litres? ☐   MEDITATION - how many minutes? ☐

SLEEP - how many hours? ☐   EXERCISE - how many minutes? ☐

LIFE EVENTS: *What happened today?*

....

....

....

EMOTIONS/THOUGHTS: *How did you feel today?*

....

....

....

CONCERNS LIST: *What bothered you most today?*

....

....

....

GRATITUDE LIST: *What are you most grateful for today?*

....

....

....

DATE .... **YEAR** ....

FOOD: *What did you eat today?*

BREAKFAST: ....

Snack: ....

LUNCH: ....

Snack: ....

DINNER: ....

Snack: ....

DRINK: *What did you drink today?*

Any caffeinated drinks: ....

Any alcoholic drinks: ....

Any other drinks: ....

Any other drugs ingested: (including prescription, recreational, over the counter and nicotine) ....

....

QUICK CHECKLIST

WATER - how many litres? ▢   MEDITATION - how many minutes? ▢

SLEEP - how many hours? ▢   EXERCISE - how many minutes? ▢

LIFE EVENTS: *What happened today?*

....

....

....

EMOTIONS/THOUGHTS: *How did you feel today?*

....

....

....

CONCERNS LIST: *What bothered you most today?*

....

....

....

GRATITUDE LIST: *What are you most grateful for today?*

....

....

....

DATE .... **YEAR** ....

FOOD: *What did you eat today?*

BREAKFAST: ....

Snack: ....

LUNCH: ....

Snack: ....

DINNER: ....

Snack: ....

DRINK: *What did you drink today?*

Any caffeinated drinks: ....

Any alcoholic drinks: ....

Any other drinks: ....

Any other drugs ingested: (including prescription, recreational, over the counter and nicotine) ....

....

QUICK CHECKLIST

WATER - how many litres? ▢   MEDITATION - how many minutes? ▢

SLEEP - how many hours? ▢   EXERCISE - how many minutes? ▢

LIFE EVENTS: *What happened today?*

....

....

....

EMOTIONS/THOUGHTS: *How did you feel today?*

....

....

....

CONCERNS LIST: *What bothered you most today?*

....

....

....

GRATITUDE LIST: *What are you most grateful for today?*

....

....

....

DATE .... **YEAR** ....

FOOD: *What did you eat today?*

BREAKFAST: ....

Snack: ....

LUNCH: ....

Snack: ....

DINNER: ....

Snack: ....

DRINK: *What did you drink today?*

Any caffeinated drinks: ....

Any alcoholic drinks: ....

Any other drinks: ....

Any other drugs ingested: (including prescription, recreational, over the counter and nicotine) ....

....

QUICK CHECKLIST

WATER - how many litres? ⬜   MEDITATION - how many minutes? ⬜

SLEEP - how many hours? ⬜   EXERCISE - how many minutes? ⬜

LIFE EVENTS: *What happened today?*

....

....

....

EMOTIONS/THOUGHTS: *How did you feel today?*

....

....

....

CONCERNS LIST: *What bothered you most today?*

....

....

....

GRATITUDE LIST: *What are you most grateful for today?*

....

....

....

DATE .... **YEAR** ....

FOOD: *What did you eat today?*

BREAKFAST: ....

Snack: ....

LUNCH: ....

Snack: ....

DINNER: ....

Snack: ....

DRINK: *What did you drink today?*

Any caffeinated drinks: ....

Any alcoholic drinks: ....

Any other drinks: ....

Any other drugs ingested: (including prescription, recreational, over the counter and nicotine) ....

....

QUICK CHECKLIST

WATER - how many litres? ☐   MEDITATION - how many minutes? ☐

SLEEP - how many hours? ☐   EXERCISE - how many minutes? ☐

LIFE EVENTS: *What happened today?*

....

....

....

EMOTIONS/THOUGHTS: *How did you feel today?*

....

....

....

CONCERNS LIST: *What bothered you most today?*

....

....

....

GRATITUDE LIST: *What are you most grateful for today?*

....

....

....

DATE .... **YEAR** ....

FOOD: *What did you eat today?*

BREAKFAST: ....

Snack: ....

LUNCH: ....

Snack: ....

DINNER: ....

Snack: ....

DRINK: *What did you drink today?*

Any caffeinated drinks: ....

Any alcoholic drinks: ....

Any other drinks: ....

Any other drugs ingested: (including prescription, recreational, over the counter and nicotine) ....

....

QUICK CHECKLIST

WATER - how many litres? ▨   MEDITATION - how many minutes? ▨

SLEEP - how many hours? ▨   EXERCISE - how many minutes? ▨

LIFE EVENTS: *What happened today?*

....

....

....

EMOTIONS/THOUGHTS: *How did you feel today?*

....

....

....

CONCERNS LIST: *What bothered you most today?*

....

....

....

GRATITUDE LIST: *What are you most grateful for today?*

....

....

....

MONTH EIGHT

alcohol

The way society views alcohol has seen a monumental shift in recent years. Dry January, Sober Spring, Dry July and Sober October - where millions of people proudly go teetotal for a month or longer - grow more popular with each passing year. Celebrities chat about rehab and recovery as candidly as they talk about their careers. Films, documentaries and TV programmes are applauded and awarded for shining a light on addiction as the serious issue that it is. Recovery websites and drinking memoirs are being published with increasing regularity and social media is awash with hashtags about addiction, sobriety and recovery all year round.

Here in the UK there's been ongoing parliamentary debate over drug law reform and recently the UK's guidelines on recommended alcohol limits were hugely reduced. Officially stating, with impressive candour that: "There is no level of regular drinking that can be considered as completely safe".

More people than ever before are looking at their relationship with alcohol. And thank goodness, because the way it's often been regarded until now has been irresponsibly dangerous. Drink misuse, abuse and dependency is a widespread, misunderstood, stigmatised pandemic health issue. Thousands of people die from it every day.

Choosing to go teetotal, for regular breaks or for good, is no longer seen as an unfortunate consequence, but as the bold, healthy, superior lifestyle choice that it is. To those people who still drink heavily and regularly, I'm not necessarily suggesting that you don't drink at all, but I am suggesting that you ask yourselves why you feel the need to drink to the extent that you do. If we're going to drink, then we must learn to drink responsibly, *truly responsibly*, every time we imbibe.

Smoking used to be promoted, endorsed and celebrated that way that alcohol often is. Alcohol is not the solution to any problem. We have to stop collectively drowning our sorrows upon hearing bad news and toasting to celebrate anything good. Our lives should not revolve around drinking alcohol, any more than they should revolve around any other drug. We must stop being so ungrateful for our precious, amazing bodies, and stop being so reckless with our lives. Our health is finite, it will not keep being renewed regardless of how shoddily we treat it. We must stop pushing our minds and our bodies to the absolute upper limits of what they can cope with, because they can't cope, not indefinitely. We no longer expect to smoke for fifty years and emerge consequence free, so why are so many of us still so casually drinking to excess?

Chugging drinks, getting sloshed, slumping, slouching and slurring all over the place is no longer viewed as an acceptable or impressive way to behave. I don't know if it ever was, but it seemed to be the norm for a long time. It's a legal, socially acceptable, mind-altering psychoactive drug that's available everywhere. Therefore it's widely used and abused by people trying to alleviate stress, anxiety, depression and boredom. Unfortunately, drinking doesn't help any of those problems in any genuine or longterm way. It only anaesthetises in the short term whilst masking the underlying problem as it contributes to it. Alcohol can create and exacerbate anxiety and depression. As an addictive substance it's easy to see why so many people develop an unhealthy relationship with it.

Slowly savouring one or two drinks with dinner on the odd occasion isn't going to cause you much harm if you're truly capable of that, but how many drinkers really do always drink like that? And do they find that sort of mindful moderation effortless? Or it is a constant exercise in controlled restriction and restraint? Only each individual person can honestly answer that for themselves. Drinking more than the recommended limit is categorically hazardous to our physical and mental health and we ignore that proven fact at our own risk. Luckily there is more fantastic help, encouragement and research available than ever before if you're struggling with a drink problem or are just plain sober curious.

So here's to the teetotallers, the sober curious, the alcohol-free serial stinters, the mindful moderators, the responsible drinkers, the abstaining 12 steppers - thanks to everyone who proves day in day out that alcohol isn't the thing that a happy healthy life revolves around. Cheers!

MONTH .... YEAR ....

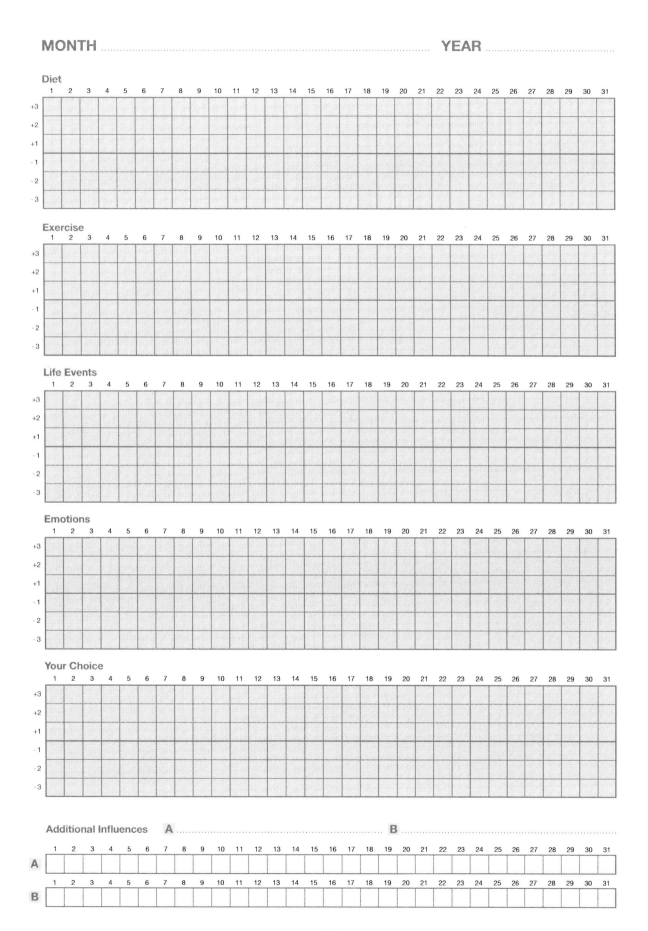

Diet

Exercise

Life Events

Emotions

Your Choice

Additional Influences A .... B ....

A

B

DATE .... **YEAR** ....

FOOD: *What did you eat today?*

BREAKFAST: ....

Snack: ....

LUNCH: ....

Snack: ....

DINNER: ....

Snack: ....

DRINK: *What did you drink today?*

Any caffeinated drinks: ....

Any alcoholic drinks: ....

Any other drinks: ....

Any other drugs ingested: (including prescription, recreational, over the counter and nicotine) ....

....

QUICK CHECKLIST

WATER - how many litres? ☐   MEDITATION - how many minutes? ☐

SLEEP - how many hours? ☐   EXERCISE - how many minutes? ☐

LIFE EVENTS: *What happened today?*

....

....

....

EMOTIONS/THOUGHTS: *How did you feel today?*

....

....

....

CONCERNS LIST: *What bothered you most today?*

....

....

....

GRATITUDE LIST: *What are you most grateful for today?*

....

....

....

DATE .... **YEAR** ....

FOOD: *What did you eat today?*

BREAKFAST: ....

Snack: ....

LUNCH: ....

Snack: ....

DINNER: ....

Snack: ....

DRINK: *What did you drink today?*

Any caffeinated drinks: ....

Any alcoholic drinks: ....

Any other drinks: ....

Any other drugs ingested: (including prescription, recreational, over the counter and nicotine) ....

....

QUICK CHECKLIST

WATER - how many litres? ▦   MEDITATION - how many minutes? ▦

SLEEP - how many hours? ▦   EXERCISE - how many minutes? ▦

LIFE EVENTS: *What happened today?*

....

....

....

EMOTIONS/THOUGHTS: *How did you feel today?*

....

....

....

CONCERNS LIST: *What bothered you most today?*

....

....

....

GRATITUDE LIST: *What are you most grateful for today?*

....

....

....

DATE .... **YEAR** ....

FOOD: *What did you eat today?*

BREAKFAST: ....

Snack: ....

LUNCH: ....

Snack: ....

DINNER: ....

Snack: ....

DRINK: *What did you drink today?*

Any caffeinated drinks: ....

Any alcoholic drinks: ....

Any other drinks: ....

Any other drugs ingested: (including prescription, recreational, over the counter and nicotine) ....

....

QUICK CHECKLIST

WATER - how many litres? ☐   MEDITATION - how many minutes? ☐

SLEEP - how many hours? ☐   EXERCISE - how many minutes? ☐

LIFE EVENTS: *What happened today?*

....

....

....

EMOTIONS/THOUGHTS: *How did you feel today?*

....

....

....

CONCERNS LIST: *What bothered you most today?*

....

....

....

GRATITUDE LIST: *What are you most grateful for today?*

....

....

....

DATE .... **YEAR** ....

FOOD: *What did you eat today?*

BREAKFAST: ....

Snack: ....

LUNCH: ....

Snack: ....

DINNER: ....

Snack: ....

DRINK: *What did you drink today?*

Any caffeinated drinks: ....

Any alcoholic drinks: ....

Any other drinks: ....

Any other drugs ingested: (including prescription, recreational, over the counter and nicotine) ....

....

QUICK CHECKLIST

WATER - how many litres? ▨   MEDITATION - how many minutes? ▨

SLEEP - how many hours? ▨   EXERCISE - how many minutes? ▨

LIFE EVENTS: *What happened today?*

....

....

....

EMOTIONS/THOUGHTS: *How did you feel today?*

....

....

....

CONCERNS LIST: *What bothered you most today?*

....

....

....

GRATITUDE LIST: *What are you most grateful for today?*

....

....

....

DATE .... **YEAR** ....

FOOD: *What did you eat today?*

BREAKFAST: ....

Snack: ....

LUNCH: ....

Snack: ....

DINNER: ....

Snack: ....

DRINK: *What did you drink today?*

Any caffeinated drinks: ....

Any alcoholic drinks: ....

Any other drinks: ....

Any other drugs ingested: (including prescription, recreational, over the counter and nicotine) ....

....

QUICK CHECKLIST

WATER - how many litres? ☐   MEDITATION - how many minutes? ☐

SLEEP - how many hours? ☐   EXERCISE - how many minutes? ☐

LIFE EVENTS: *What happened today?*

....

....

....

EMOTIONS/THOUGHTS: *How did you feel today?*

....

....

....

CONCERNS LIST: *What bothered you most today?*

....

....

....

GRATITUDE LIST: *What are you most grateful for today?*

....

....

....

DATE .... **YEAR** ....

FOOD: *What did you eat today?*

BREAKFAST: ....

Snack: ....

LUNCH: ....

Snack: ....

DINNER: ....

Snack: ....

DRINK: *What did you drink today?*

Any caffeinated drinks: ....

Any alcoholic drinks: ....

Any other drinks: ....

Any other drugs ingested: (including prescription, recreational, over the counter and nicotine) ....

....

QUICK CHECKLIST

WATER - how many litres? ▨   MEDITATION - how many minutes? ▨

SLEEP - how many hours? ▨   EXERCISE - how many minutes? ▨

LIFE EVENTS: *What happened today?*

....

....

....

EMOTIONS/THOUGHTS: *How did you feel today?*

....

....

....

CONCERNS LIST: *What bothered you most today?*

....

....

....

GRATITUDE LIST: *What are you most grateful for today?*

....

....

....

DATE .... **YEAR** ....

FOOD: *What did you eat today?*

BREAKFAST: ....

Snack: ....

LUNCH: ....

Snack: ....

DINNER: ....

Snack: ....

DRINK: *What did you drink today?*

Any caffeinated drinks: ....

Any alcoholic drinks: ....

Any other drinks: ....

Any other drugs ingested: (including prescription, recreational, over the counter and nicotine) ....

....

QUICK CHECKLIST

WATER - how many litres? ▢   MEDITATION - how many minutes? ▢

SLEEP - how many hours? ▢   EXERCISE - how many minutes? ▢

LIFE EVENTS: *What happened today?*

....

....

....

EMOTIONS/THOUGHTS: *How did you feel today?*

....

....

....

CONCERNS LIST: *What bothered you most today?*

....

....

....

GRATITUDE LIST: *What are you most grateful for today?*

....

....

....

DATE .... **YEAR** ....

FOOD: *What did you eat today?*

BREAKFAST: ....

Snack: ....

LUNCH: ....

Snack: ....

DINNER: ....

Snack: ....

DRINK: *What did you drink today?*

Any caffeinated drinks: ....

Any alcoholic drinks: ....

Any other drinks: ....

Any other drugs ingested: (including prescription, recreational, over the counter and nicotine) ....

....

QUICK CHECKLIST

WATER - how many litres? ▦   MEDITATION - how many minutes? ▦

SLEEP - how many hours? ▦   EXERCISE - how many minutes? ▦

LIFE EVENTS: *What happened today?*

....

....

....

EMOTIONS/THOUGHTS: *How did you feel today?*

....

....

....

CONCERNS LIST: *What bothered you most today?*

....

....

....

GRATITUDE LIST: *What are you most grateful for today?*

....

....

....

DATE .... **YEAR** ....

FOOD: *What did you eat today?*

BREAKFAST: ....

Snack: ....

LUNCH: ....

Snack: ....

DINNER: ....

Snack: ....

DRINK: *What did you drink today?*

Any caffeinated drinks: ....

Any alcoholic drinks: ....

Any other drinks: ....

Any other drugs ingested: (including prescription, recreational, over the counter and nicotine) ....

....

QUICK CHECKLIST

WATER - how many litres? ☐   MEDITATION - how many minutes? ☐

SLEEP - how many hours? ☐   EXERCISE - how many minutes? ☐

LIFE EVENTS: *What happened today?*

....

....

....

EMOTIONS/THOUGHTS: *How did you feel today?*

....

....

....

CONCERNS LIST: *What bothered you most today?*

....

....

....

GRATITUDE LIST: *What are you most grateful for today?*

....

....

....

DATE .... **YEAR** ....

FOOD: *What did you eat today?*

BREAKFAST: ....

Snack: ....

LUNCH: ....

Snack: ....

DINNER: ....

Snack: ....

DRINK: *What did you drink today?*

Any caffeinated drinks: ....

Any alcoholic drinks: ....

Any other drinks: ....

Any other drugs ingested: (including prescription, recreational, over the counter and nicotine) ....

....

QUICK CHECKLIST

WATER - how many litres? ▨   MEDITATION - how many minutes? ▨

SLEEP - how many hours? ▨   EXERCISE - how many minutes? ▨

LIFE EVENTS: *What happened today?*

....

....

....

EMOTIONS/THOUGHTS: *How did you feel today?*

....

....

....

CONCERNS LIST: *What bothered you most today?*

....

....

....

GRATITUDE LIST: *What are you most grateful for today?*

....

....

....

DATE .... **YEAR** ....

FOOD: *What did you eat today?*

BREAKFAST: ....

Snack: ....

LUNCH: ....

Snack: ....

DINNER: ....

Snack: ....

DRINK: *What did you drink today?*

Any caffeinated drinks: ....

Any alcoholic drinks: ....

Any other drinks: ....

Any other drugs ingested: (including prescription, recreational, over the counter and nicotine) ....

....

QUICK CHECKLIST

WATER - how many litres? ☐   MEDITATION - how many minutes? ☐

SLEEP - how many hours? ☐   EXERCISE - how many minutes? ☐

LIFE EVENTS: *What happened today?*

....

....

....

EMOTIONS/THOUGHTS: *How did you feel today?*

....

....

....

CONCERNS LIST: *What bothered you most today?*

....

....

....

GRATITUDE LIST: *What are you most grateful for today?*

....

....

....

DATE .... **YEAR** ....

FOOD: *What did you eat today?*

BREAKFAST: ....

Snack: ....

LUNCH: ....

Snack: ....

DINNER: ....

Snack: ....

DRINK: *What did you drink today?*

Any caffeinated drinks: ....

Any alcoholic drinks: ....

Any other drinks: ....

Any other drugs ingested: (including prescription, recreational, over the counter and nicotine) ....

....

QUICK CHECKLIST

WATER - how many litres? ▢   MEDITATION - how many minutes? ▢

SLEEP - how many hours? ▢   EXERCISE - how many minutes? ▢

LIFE EVENTS: *What happened today?*

....

....

....

EMOTIONS/THOUGHTS: *How did you feel today?*

....

....

....

CONCERNS LIST: *What bothered you most today?*

....

....

....

GRATITUDE LIST: *What are you most grateful for today?*

....

....

....

DATE .... **YEAR** ....

FOOD: *What did you eat today?*

BREAKFAST: ....

Snack: ....

LUNCH: ....

Snack: ....

DINNER: ....

Snack: ....

DRINK: *What did you drink today?*

Any caffeinated drinks: ....

Any alcoholic drinks: ....

Any other drinks: ....

Any other drugs ingested: (including prescription, recreational, over the counter and nicotine) ....

....

QUICK CHECKLIST

WATER - how many litres? ☐   MEDITATION - how many minutes? ☐

SLEEP - how many hours? ☐   EXERCISE - how many minutes? ☐

LIFE EVENTS: *What happened today?*

....

....

....

EMOTIONS/THOUGHTS: *How did you feel today?*

....

....

....

CONCERNS LIST: *What bothered you most today?*

....

....

....

GRATITUDE LIST: *What are you most grateful for today?*

....

....

....

DATE .... **YEAR** ....

FOOD: *What did you eat today?*

BREAKFAST: ....

Snack: ....

LUNCH: ....

Snack: ....

DINNER: ....

Snack: ....

DRINK: *What did you drink today?*

Any caffeinated drinks: ....

Any alcoholic drinks: ....

Any other drinks: ....

Any other drugs ingested: (including prescription, recreational, over the counter and nicotine) ....

....

QUICK CHECKLIST

WATER - how many litres? ▢   MEDITATION - how many minutes? ▢

SLEEP - how many hours? ▢   EXERCISE - how many minutes? ▢

LIFE EVENTS: *What happened today?*

....

....

....

EMOTIONS/THOUGHTS: *How did you feel today?*

....

....

....

CONCERNS LIST: *What bothered you most today?*

....

....

....

GRATITUDE LIST: *What are you most grateful for today?*

....

....

....

DATE .... **YEAR** ....

FOOD: *What did you eat today?*

BREAKFAST: ....

Snack: ....

LUNCH: ....

Snack: ....

DINNER: ....

Snack: ....

DRINK: *What did you drink today?*

Any caffeinated drinks: ....

Any alcoholic drinks: ....

Any other drinks: ....

Any other drugs ingested: (including prescription, recreational, over the counter and nicotine) ....

....

QUICK CHECKLIST

WATER - how many litres? ▢   MEDITATION - how many minutes? ▢

SLEEP - how many hours? ▢   EXERCISE - how many minutes? ▢

LIFE EVENTS: *What happened today?*

....

....

....

EMOTIONS/THOUGHTS: *How did you feel today?*

....

....

....

CONCERNS LIST: *What bothered you most today?*

....

....

....

GRATITUDE LIST: *What are you most grateful for today?*

....

....

....

DATE .... **YEAR** ....

FOOD: *What did you eat today?*

BREAKFAST: ....

Snack: ....

LUNCH: ....

Snack: ....

DINNER: ....

Snack: ....

DRINK: *What did you drink today?*

Any caffeinated drinks: ....

Any alcoholic drinks: ....

Any other drinks: ....

Any other drugs ingested: (including prescription, recreational, over the counter and nicotine) ....

....

QUICK CHECKLIST

WATER - how many litres? ▨   MEDITATION - how many minutes? ▨

SLEEP - how many hours? ▨   EXERCISE - how many minutes? ▨

LIFE EVENTS: *What happened today?*

....

....

....

EMOTIONS/THOUGHTS: *How did you feel today?*

....

....

....

CONCERNS LIST: *What bothered you most today?*

....

....

....

GRATITUDE LIST: *What are you most grateful for today?*

....

....

....

DATE .... **YEAR** ....

FOOD: *What did you eat today?*

BREAKFAST: ....

Snack: ....

LUNCH: ....

Snack: ....

DINNER: ....

Snack: ....

DRINK: *What did you drink today?*

Any caffeinated drinks: ....

Any alcoholic drinks: ....

Any other drinks: ....

Any other drugs ingested: (including prescription, recreational, over the counter and nicotine) ....
....

QUICK CHECKLIST

WATER - how many litres? ☐   MEDITATION - how many minutes? ☐

SLEEP - how many hours? ☐   EXERCISE - how many minutes? ☐

LIFE EVENTS: *What happened today?*

....
....
....

EMOTIONS/THOUGHTS: *How did you feel today?*

....
....
....

CONCERNS LIST: *What bothered you most today?*

....
....
....

GRATITUDE LIST: *What are you most grateful for today?*

....
....
....

DATE .... **YEAR** ....

FOOD: *What did you eat today?*

BREAKFAST: ....

Snack: ....

LUNCH: ....

Snack: ....

DINNER: ....

Snack: ....

DRINK: *What did you drink today?*

Any caffeinated drinks: ....

Any alcoholic drinks: ....

Any other drinks: ....

Any other drugs ingested: (including prescription, recreational, over the counter and nicotine) ....

....

QUICK CHECKLIST

WATER - how many litres? ☐   MEDITATION - how many minutes? ☐

SLEEP - how many hours? ☐   EXERCISE - how many minutes? ☐

LIFE EVENTS: *What happened today?*

....

....

....

EMOTIONS/THOUGHTS: *How did you feel today?*

....

....

....

CONCERNS LIST: *What bothered you most today?*

....

....

....

GRATITUDE LIST: *What are you most grateful for today?*

....

....

....

DATE .... YEAR ....

FOOD: *What did you eat today?*

BREAKFAST: ....

Snack: ....

LUNCH: ....

Snack: ....

DINNER: ....

Snack: ....

DRINK: *What did you drink today?*

Any caffeinated drinks: ....

Any alcoholic drinks: ....

Any other drinks: ....

Any other drugs ingested: (including prescription, recreational, over the counter and nicotine) ....

....

QUICK CHECKLIST

WATER - how many litres? ☐   MEDITATION - how many minutes? ☐

SLEEP - how many hours? ☐   EXERCISE - how many minutes? ☐

LIFE EVENTS: *What happened today?*

....

....

....

EMOTIONS/THOUGHTS: *How did you feel today?*

....

....

....

CONCERNS LIST: *What bothered you most today?*

....

....

....

GRATITUDE LIST: *What are you most grateful for today?*

....

....

....

DATE .... YEAR ....

FOOD: *What did you eat today?*

BREAKFAST: ....

Snack: ....

LUNCH: ....

Snack: ....

DINNER: ....

Snack: ....

DRINK: *What did you drink today?*

Any caffeinated drinks: ....

Any alcoholic drinks: ....

Any other drinks: ....

Any other drugs ingested: (including prescription, recreational, over the counter and nicotine) ....

....

QUICK CHECKLIST

WATER - how many litres? ▢   MEDITATION - how many minutes? ▢

SLEEP - how many hours? ▢   EXERCISE - how many minutes? ▢

LIFE EVENTS: *What happened today?*

....

....

....

EMOTIONS/THOUGHTS: *How did you feel today?*

....

....

....

CONCERNS LIST: *What bothered you most today?*

....

....

....

GRATITUDE LIST: *What are you most grateful for today?*

....

....

....

DATE .... YEAR ....

FOOD: *What did you eat today?*

BREAKFAST: ....

Snack: ....

LUNCH: ....

Snack: ....

DINNER: ....

Snack: ....

DRINK: *What did you drink today?*

Any caffeinated drinks: ....

Any alcoholic drinks: ....

Any other drinks: ....

Any other drugs ingested: (including prescription, recreational, over the counter and nicotine) ....

....

QUICK CHECKLIST

WATER - how many litres? ☐   MEDITATION - how many minutes? ☐

SLEEP - how many hours? ☐   EXERCISE - how many minutes? ☐

LIFE EVENTS: *What happened today?*

....

....

....

EMOTIONS/THOUGHTS: *How did you feel today?*

....

....

....

CONCERNS LIST: *What bothered you most today?*

....

....

....

GRATITUDE LIST: *What are you most grateful for today?*

....

....

....

DATE .... YEAR ....

FOOD: *What did you eat today?*

BREAKFAST: ....

Snack: ....

LUNCH: ....

Snack: ....

DINNER: ....

Snack: ....

DRINK: *What did you drink today?*

Any caffeinated drinks: ....

Any alcoholic drinks: ....

Any other drinks: ....

Any other drugs ingested: (including prescription, recreational, over the counter and nicotine) ....

....

QUICK CHECKLIST

WATER - how many litres? ▨   MEDITATION - how many minutes? ▨

SLEEP - how many hours? ▨   EXERCISE - how many minutes? ▨

LIFE EVENTS: *What happened today?*

....

....

....

EMOTIONS/THOUGHTS: *How did you feel today?*

....

....

....

CONCERNS LIST: *What bothered you most today?*

....

....

....

GRATITUDE LIST: *What are you most grateful for today?*

....

....

....

DATE .... **YEAR** ....

FOOD: *What did you eat today?*

BREAKFAST: ....

Snack: ....

LUNCH: ....

Snack: ....

DINNER: ....

Snack: ....

DRINK: *What did you drink today?*

Any caffeinated drinks: ....

Any alcoholic drinks: ....

Any other drinks: ....

Any other drugs ingested: (including prescription, recreational, over the counter and nicotine) ....

....

QUICK CHECKLIST

WATER - how many litres? ☐   MEDITATION - how many minutes? ☐

SLEEP - how many hours? ☐   EXERCISE - how many minutes? ☐

LIFE EVENTS: *What happened today?*

....

....

....

EMOTIONS/THOUGHTS: *How did you feel today?*

....

....

....

CONCERNS LIST: *What bothered you most today?*

....

....

....

GRATITUDE LIST: *What are you most grateful for today?*

....

....

....

DATE .... **YEAR** ....

FOOD: *What did you eat today?*

BREAKFAST: ....

Snack: ....

LUNCH: ....

Snack: ....

DINNER: ....

Snack: ....

DRINK: *What did you drink today?*

Any caffeinated drinks: ....

Any alcoholic drinks: ....

Any other drinks: ....

Any other drugs ingested: (including prescription, recreational, over the counter and nicotine) ....

....

QUICK CHECKLIST

WATER - how many litres? ▨   MEDITATION - how many minutes? ▨

SLEEP - how many hours? ▨   EXERCISE - how many minutes? ▨

LIFE EVENTS: *What happened today?*

....

....

....

EMOTIONS/THOUGHTS: *How did you feel today?*

....

....

....

CONCERNS LIST: *What bothered you most today?*

....

....

....

GRATITUDE LIST: *What are you most grateful for today?*

....

....

....

DATE .... **YEAR** ....

FOOD: *What did you eat today?*

BREAKFAST: ....

Snack: ....

LUNCH: ....

Snack: ....

DINNER: ....

Snack: ....

DRINK: *What did you drink today?*

Any caffeinated drinks: ....

Any alcoholic drinks: ....

Any other drinks: ....

Any other drugs ingested: (including prescription, recreational, over the counter and nicotine) ....

....

QUICK CHECKLIST

WATER - how many litres? ☐   MEDITATION - how many minutes? ☐

SLEEP - how many hours? ☐   EXERCISE - how many minutes? ☐

LIFE EVENTS: *What happened today?*

....

....

....

EMOTIONS/THOUGHTS: *How did you feel today?*

....

....

....

CONCERNS LIST: *What bothered you most today?*

....

....

....

GRATITUDE LIST: *What are you most grateful for today?*

....

....

....

DATE .... **YEAR** ....

FOOD: *What did you eat today?*

BREAKFAST: ....

Snack: ....

LUNCH: ....

Snack: ....

DINNER: ....

Snack: ....

DRINK: *What did you drink today?*

Any caffeinated drinks: ....

Any alcoholic drinks: ....

Any other drinks: ....

Any other drugs ingested: (including prescription, recreational, over the counter and nicotine) ....

....

QUICK CHECKLIST

WATER - how many litres? ▦   MEDITATION - how many minutes? ▦

SLEEP - how many hours? ▦   EXERCISE - how many minutes? ▦

LIFE EVENTS: *What happened today?*

....

....

....

EMOTIONS/THOUGHTS: *How did you feel today?*

....

....

....

CONCERNS LIST: *What bothered you most today?*

....

....

....

GRATITUDE LIST: *What are you most grateful for today?*

....

....

....

DATE .... **YEAR** ....

FOOD: *What did you eat today?*

BREAKFAST: ....

Snack: ....

LUNCH: ....

Snack: ....

DINNER: ....

Snack: ....

DRINK: *What did you drink today?*

Any caffeinated drinks: ....

Any alcoholic drinks: ....

Any other drinks: ....

Any other drugs ingested: (including prescription, recreational, over the counter and nicotine) ....

....

QUICK CHECKLIST

WATER - how many litres? ▢   MEDITATION - how many minutes? ▢

SLEEP - how many hours? ▢   EXERCISE - how many minutes? ▢

LIFE EVENTS: *What happened today?*

....

....

....

EMOTIONS/THOUGHTS: *How did you feel today?*

....

....

....

CONCERNS LIST: *What bothered you most today?*

....

....

....

GRATITUDE LIST: *What are you most grateful for today?*

....

....

....

DATE .... **YEAR** ....

FOOD: *What did you eat today?*

BREAKFAST: ....

Snack: ....

LUNCH: ....

Snack: ....

DINNER: ....

Snack: ....

DRINK: *What did you drink today?*

Any caffeinated drinks: ....

Any alcoholic drinks: ....

Any other drinks: ....

Any other drugs ingested: (including prescription, recreational, over the counter and nicotine) ....

....

QUICK CHECKLIST

WATER - how many litres? ☐   MEDITATION - how many minutes? ☐

SLEEP - how many hours? ☐   EXERCISE - how many minutes? ☐

LIFE EVENTS: *What happened today?*

....

....

....

EMOTIONS/THOUGHTS: *How did you feel today?*

....

....

....

CONCERNS LIST: *What bothered you most today?*

....

....

....

GRATITUDE LIST: *What are you most grateful for today?*

....

....

....

DATE .... **YEAR** ....

FOOD: *What did you eat today?*

BREAKFAST: ....

Snack: ....

LUNCH: ....

Snack: ....

DINNER: ....

Snack: ....

DRINK: *What did you drink today?*

Any caffeinated drinks: ....

Any alcoholic drinks: ....

Any other drinks: ....

Any other drugs ingested: (including prescription, recreational, over the counter and nicotine) ....
....

QUICK CHECKLIST

WATER - how many litres? ▢   MEDITATION - how many minutes? ▢

SLEEP - how many hours? ▢   EXERCISE - how many minutes? ▢

LIFE EVENTS: *What happened today?*

....

....

....

EMOTIONS/THOUGHTS: *How did you feel today?*

....

....

....

CONCERNS LIST: *What bothered you most today?*

....

....

....

GRATITUDE LIST: *What are you most grateful for today?*

....

....

....

DATE .... **YEAR** ....

FOOD: *What did you eat today?*

BREAKFAST: ....

Snack: ....

LUNCH: ....

Snack: ....

DINNER: ....

Snack: ....

DRINK: *What did you drink today?*

Any caffeinated drinks: ....

Any alcoholic drinks: ....

Any other drinks: ....

Any other drugs ingested: (including prescription, recreational, over the counter and nicotine) ....

....

QUICK CHECKLIST

WATER - how many litres? ▢   MEDITATION - how many minutes? ▢

SLEEP - how many hours? ▢   EXERCISE - how many minutes? ▢

LIFE EVENTS: *What happened today?*

....

....

....

EMOTIONS/THOUGHTS: *How did you feel today?*

....

....

....

CONCERNS LIST: *What bothered you most today?*

....

....

....

GRATITUDE LIST: *What are you most grateful for today?*

....

....

....

DATE .... **YEAR** ....

FOOD: *What did you eat today?*

BREAKFAST: ....

Snack: ....

LUNCH: ....

Snack: ....

DINNER: ....

Snack: ....

DRINK: *What did you drink today?*

Any caffeinated drinks: ....

Any alcoholic drinks: ....

Any other drinks: ....

Any other drugs ingested: (including prescription, recreational, over the counter and nicotine) ....

....

QUICK CHECKLIST

WATER - how many litres? ▨   MEDITATION - how many minutes? ▨

SLEEP - how many hours? ▨   EXERCISE - how many minutes? ▨

LIFE EVENTS: *What happened today?*

....

....

....

EMOTIONS/THOUGHTS: *How did you feel today?*

....

....

....

CONCERNS LIST: *What bothered you most today?*

....

....

....

GRATITUDE LIST: *What are you most grateful for today?*

....

....

....

MONTH

NINE

<u>patience and motivation</u>

If you fully commit to using this journal, you will definitely see patterns emerge and you will be able to make changes for the better, but only as a result of your efforts, your mindful, consistent, daily discipline. (This is often the best way to make long-lasting lifestyle changes; in sure-footed incremental steps, rather than by a sudden shock to the system.)

Small manageable efforts made day in, day out add up to enormous results over the course of a whole year. If you keep putting the work in, day after day, honestly tracking your progress and learning as you grow - you can't fail to see results.

Always keep your focus predominantly on where you are right now and what you'll do next, to move you that little bit closer to your goals. We don't live in the past or in the future and so we can't control what happened/happens there. We live in the moment, in the perpetual present, and so it's always your very next decision that's the most important one. What you do today will directly affect tomorrow. Have patience and stay safely rooted in the present moment and your future will take care of itself.

The art of cultivating poise and patience is necessary in order to lead a healthy well-balanced life. We will all experience ups and downs, the quiet calms and the scary storms. A cool persever-ance, especially in times of stress and struggle, is exactly what will allow you the freedom to hold onto your resolve. It doesn't do anybody any good to abandon their commitments during times of unease. In fact, in times of discomfort, that's when we need to hold on even more tightly to our hopes and dreams, and self-care routines, and the knowledge that we are always accountable for our own choices, whether we're in the calm or in the storm.

The more patience you cultivate, the better results you'll see, and the more motivation you'll feel. And just like magic, one glorious day, you'll notice how new habits have sprung up in place of the old ones and you'll suddenly realise that you were strong enough to do this all along. You were just weighed down before, and now you're not. Now, you can do better, because you know better.

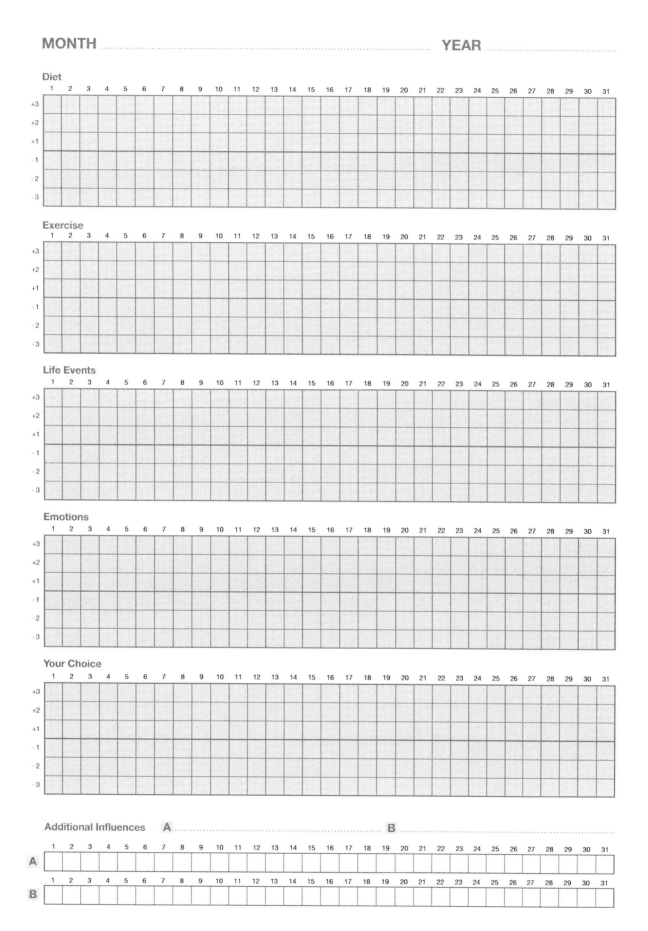

MONTH .... YEAR ....

Diet

Exercise

Life Events

Emotions

Your Choice

Additional Influences A .... B ....

DATE .... **YEAR** ....

FOOD: *What did you eat today?*

BREAKFAST: ....

Snack: ....

LUNCH: ....

Snack: ....

DINNER: ....

Snack: ....

DRINK: *What did you drink today?*

Any caffeinated drinks: ....

Any alcoholic drinks: ....

Any other drinks: ....

Any other drugs ingested: (including prescription, recreational, over the counter and nicotine) ....

....

QUICK CHECKLIST

WATER - how many litres? ▢   MEDITATION - how many minutes? ▢

SLEEP - how many hours? ▢   EXERCISE - how many minutes? ▢

LIFE EVENTS: *What happened today?*

....

....

....

EMOTIONS/THOUGHTS: *How did you feel today?*

....

....

....

CONCERNS LIST: *What bothered you most today?*

....

....

....

GRATITUDE LIST: *What are you most grateful for today?*

....

....

....

DATE .... **YEAR** ....

FOOD: *What did you eat today?*

BREAKFAST: ....

Snack: ....

LUNCH: ....

Snack: ....

DINNER: ....

Snack: ....

DRINK: *What did you drink today?*

Any caffeinated drinks: ....

Any alcoholic drinks: ....

Any other drinks: ....

Any other drugs ingested: (including prescription, recreational, over the counter and nicotine) ....

....

QUICK CHECKLIST

WATER - how many litres? ▨   MEDITATION - how many minutes? ▨

SLEEP - how many hours? ▨   EXERCISE - how many minutes? ▨

LIFE EVENTS: *What happened today?*

....

....

....

EMOTIONS/THOUGHTS: *How did you feel today?*

....

....

....

CONCERNS LIST: *What bothered you most today?*

....

....

....

GRATITUDE LIST: *What are you most grateful for today?*

....

....

....

DATE .... **YEAR** ....

FOOD: *What did you eat today?*

BREAKFAST: ....

Snack: ....

LUNCH: ....

Snack: ....

DINNER: ....

Snack: ....

DRINK: *What did you drink today?*

Any caffeinated drinks: ....

Any alcoholic drinks: ....

Any other drinks: ....

Any other drugs ingested: (including prescription, recreational, over the counter and nicotine) ....

....

QUICK CHECKLIST

WATER - how many litres? ☐   MEDITATION - how many minutes? ☐

SLEEP - how many hours? ☐   EXERCISE - how many minutes? ☐

LIFE EVENTS: *What happened today?*

....

....

....

EMOTIONS/THOUGHTS: *How did you feel today?*

....

....

....

CONCERNS LIST: *What bothered you most today?*

....

....

....

GRATITUDE LIST: *What are you most grateful for today?*

....

....

....

DATE .... **YEAR** ....

FOOD: *What did you eat today?*

BREAKFAST: ....

Snack: ....

LUNCH: ....

Snack: ....

DINNER: ....

Snack: ....

DRINK: *What did you drink today?*

Any caffeinated drinks: ....

Any alcoholic drinks: ....

Any other drinks: ....

Any other drugs ingested: (including prescription, recreational, over the counter and nicotine) ....

....

QUICK CHECKLIST

WATER - how many litres? ▨   MEDITATION - how many minutes? ▨

SLEEP - how many hours? ▨   EXERCISE - how many minutes? ▨

LIFE EVENTS: *What happened today?*

....

....

....

EMOTIONS/THOUGHTS: *How did you feel today?*

....

....

....

CONCERNS LIST: *What bothered you most today?*

....

....

....

GRATITUDE LIST: *What are you most grateful for today?*

....

....

....

DATE .... **YEAR** ....

FOOD: *What did you eat today?*

BREAKFAST: ....

Snack: ....

LUNCH: ....

Snack: ....

DINNER: ....

Snack: ....

DRINK: *What did you drink today?*

Any caffeinated drinks: ....

Any alcoholic drinks: ....

Any other drinks: ....

Any other drugs ingested: (including prescription, recreational, over the counter and nicotine) ....

....

QUICK CHECKLIST

WATER - how many litres? ▢   MEDITATION - how many minutes? ▢

SLEEP - how many hours? ▢   EXERCISE - how many minutes? ▢

LIFE EVENTS: *What happened today?*

....

....

....

EMOTIONS/THOUGHTS: *How did you feel today?*

....

....

....

CONCERNS LIST: *What bothered you most today?*

....

....

....

GRATITUDE LIST: *What are you most grateful for today?*

....

....

....

DATE .... **YEAR** ....

FOOD: *What did you eat today?*

BREAKFAST: ....

Snack: ....

LUNCH: ....

Snack: ....

DINNER: ....

Snack: ....

DRINK: *What did you drink today?*

Any caffeinated drinks: ....

Any alcoholic drinks: ....

Any other drinks: ....

Any other drugs ingested: (including prescription, recreational, over the counter and nicotine) ....

....

QUICK CHECKLIST

WATER - how many litres? ▓   MEDITATION - how many minutes? ▓

SLEEP - how many hours? ▓   EXERCISE - how many minutes? ▓

LIFE EVENTS: *What happened today?*

....

....

....

EMOTIONS/THOUGHTS: *How did you feel today?*

....

....

....

CONCERNS LIST: *What bothered you most today?*

....

....

....

GRATITUDE LIST: *What are you most grateful for today?*

....

....

....

DATE .... **YEAR** ....

FOOD: *What did you eat today?*

BREAKFAST: ....

Snack: ....

LUNCH: ....

Snack: ....

DINNER: ....

Snack: ....

DRINK: *What did you drink today?*

Any caffeinated drinks: ....

Any alcoholic drinks: ....

Any other drinks: ....

Any other drugs ingested: (including prescription, recreational, over the counter and nicotine) ....

....

QUICK CHECKLIST

WATER - how many litres? ▢   MEDITATION - how many minutes? ▢

SLEEP - how many hours? ▢   EXERCISE - how many minutes? ▢

LIFE EVENTS: *What happened today?*

....

....

....

EMOTIONS/THOUGHTS: *How did you feel today?*

....

....

....

CONCERNS LIST: *What bothered you most today?*

....

....

....

GRATITUDE LIST: *What are you most grateful for today?*

....

....

....

DATE .... **YEAR** ....

FOOD: *What did you eat today?*

BREAKFAST: ....

Snack: ....

LUNCH: ....

Snack: ....

DINNER: ....

Snack: ....

DRINK: *What did you drink today?*

Any caffeinated drinks: ....

Any alcoholic drinks: ....

Any other drinks: ....

Any other drugs ingested: (including prescription, recreational, over the counter and nicotine) ....

....

QUICK CHECKLIST

WATER - how many litres? ▨   MEDITATION - how many minutes? ▨

SLEEP - how many hours? ▨   EXERCISE - how many minutes? ▨

LIFE EVENTS: *What happened today?*

....

....

....

EMOTIONS/THOUGHTS: *How did you feel today?*

....

....

....

CONCERNS LIST: *What bothered you most today?*

....

....

....

GRATITUDE LIST: *What are you most grateful for today?*

....

....

....

DATE .... **YEAR** ....

FOOD: *What did you eat today?*

BREAKFAST: ....

Snack: ....

LUNCH: ....

Snack: ....

DINNER: ....

Snack: ....

DRINK: *What did you drink today?*

Any caffeinated drinks: ....

Any alcoholic drinks: ....

Any other drinks: ....

Any other drugs ingested: (including prescription, recreational, over the counter and nicotine) ....

....

QUICK CHECKLIST

WATER - how many litres? ▨   MEDITATION - how many minutes? ▨

SLEEP - how many hours? ▨   EXERCISE - how many minutes? ▨

LIFE EVENTS: *What happened today?*

....

....

....

EMOTIONS/THOUGHTS: *How did you feel today?*

....

....

....

CONCERNS LIST: *What bothered you most today?*

....

....

....

GRATITUDE LIST: *What are you most grateful for today?*

....

....

....

DATE .... **YEAR** ....

FOOD: *What did you eat today?*

BREAKFAST: ....

Snack: ....

LUNCH: ....

Snack: ....

DINNER: ....

Snack: ....

DRINK: *What did you drink today?*

Any caffeinated drinks: ....

Any alcoholic drinks: ....

Any other drinks: ....

Any other drugs ingested: (including prescription, recreational, over the counter and nicotine) ....

....

QUICK CHECKLIST

WATER - how many litres? ▪   MEDITATION - how many minutes? ▪

SLEEP - how many hours? ▪   EXERCISE - how many minutes? ▪

LIFE EVENTS: *What happened today?*

....

....

....

EMOTIONS/THOUGHTS: *How did you feel today?*

....

....

....

CONCERNS LIST: *What bothered you most today?*

....

....

....

GRATITUDE LIST: *What are you most grateful for today?*

....

....

....

DATE .... **YEAR** ....

FOOD: *What did you eat today?*

BREAKFAST: ....

Snack: ....

LUNCH: ....

Snack: ....

DINNER: ....

Snack: ....

DRINK: *What did you drink today?*

Any caffeinated drinks: ....

Any alcoholic drinks: ....

Any other drinks: ....

Any other drugs ingested: (including prescription, recreational, over the counter and nicotine) ....

....

QUICK CHECKLIST

WATER - how many litres? ▢   MEDITATION - how many minutes? ▢

SLEEP - how many hours? ▢   EXERCISE - how many minutes? ▢

LIFE EVENTS: *What happened today?*

....

....

....

EMOTIONS/THOUGHTS: *How did you feel today?*

....

....

....

CONCERNS LIST: *What bothered you most today?*

....

....

....

GRATITUDE LIST: *What are you most grateful for today?*

....

....

....

DATE .... **YEAR** ....

FOOD: *What did you eat today?*

BREAKFAST: ....

Snack: ....

LUNCH: ....

Snack: ....

DINNER: ....

Snack: ....

DRINK: *What did you drink today?*

Any caffeinated drinks: ....

Any alcoholic drinks: ....

Any other drinks: ....

Any other drugs ingested: (including prescription, recreational, over the counter and nicotine) ....

....

QUICK CHECKLIST

WATER - how many litres? ☐   MEDITATION - how many minutes? ☐

SLEEP - how many hours? ☐   EXERCISE - how many minutes? ☐

LIFE EVENTS: *What happened today?*

....

....

....

EMOTIONS/THOUGHTS: *How did you feel today?*

....

....

....

CONCERNS LIST: *What bothered you most today?*

....

....

....

GRATITUDE LIST: *What are you most grateful for today?*

....

....

....

DATE .... **YEAR** ....

FOOD: *What did you eat today?*

BREAKFAST: ....

Snack: ....

LUNCH: ....

Snack: ....

DINNER: ....

Snack: ....

DRINK: *What did you drink today?*

Any caffeinated drinks: ....

Any alcoholic drinks: ....

Any other drinks: ....

Any other drugs ingested: (including prescription, recreational, over the counter and nicotine) ....

....

QUICK CHECKLIST

WATER - how many litres? ☐   MEDITATION - how many minutes? ☐

SLEEP - how many hours? ☐   EXERCISE - how many minutes? ☐

LIFE EVENTS: *What happened today?*

....

....

....

EMOTIONS/THOUGHTS: *How did you feel today?*

....

....

....

CONCERNS LIST: *What bothered you most today?*

....

....

....

GRATITUDE LIST: *What are you most grateful for today?*

....

....

....

DATE .... **YEAR** ....

FOOD: *What did you eat today?*

BREAKFAST: ....

Snack: ....

LUNCH: ....

Snack: ....

DINNER: ....

Snack: ....

DRINK: *What did you drink today?*

Any caffeinated drinks: ....

Any alcoholic drinks: ....

Any other drinks: ....

Any other drugs ingested: (including prescription, recreational, over the counter and nicotine) ....

....

QUICK CHECKLIST

WATER - how many litres? ▨   MEDITATION - how many minutes? ▨

SLEEP - how many hours? ▨   EXERCISE - how many minutes? ▨

LIFE EVENTS: *What happened today?*

....

....

....

EMOTIONS/THOUGHTS: *How did you feel today?*

....

....

....

CONCERNS LIST: *What bothered you most today?*

....

....

....

GRATITUDE LIST: *What are you most grateful for today?*

....

....

....

DATE .... **YEAR** ....

FOOD: *What did you eat today?*

BREAKFAST: ....

Snack: ....

LUNCH: ....

Snack: ....

DINNER: ....

Snack: ....

DRINK: *What did you drink today?*

Any caffeinated drinks: ....

Any alcoholic drinks: ....

Any other drinks: ....

Any other drugs ingested: (including prescription, recreational, over the counter and nicotine) ....

....

QUICK CHECKLIST

WATER - how many litres? ☐   MEDITATION - how many minutes? ☐

SLEEP - how many hours? ☐   EXERCISE - how many minutes? ☐

LIFE EVENTS: *What happened today?*

....

....

....

EMOTIONS/THOUGHTS: *How did you feel today?*

....

....

....

CONCERNS LIST: *What bothered you most today?*

....

....

....

GRATITUDE LIST: *What are you most grateful for today?*

....

....

....

DATE .... **YEAR** ....

FOOD: *What did you eat today?*

BREAKFAST: ....

Snack: ....

LUNCH: ....

Snack: ....

DINNER: ....

Snack: ....

DRINK: *What did you drink today?*

Any caffeinated drinks: ....

Any alcoholic drinks: ....

Any other drinks: ....

Any other drugs ingested: (including prescription, recreational, over the counter and nicotine) ....

....

QUICK CHECKLIST

WATER - how many litres? ▨   MEDITATION - how many minutes? ▨

SLEEP - how many hours? ▨   EXERCISE - how many minutes? ▨

LIFE EVENTS: *What happened today?*

....

....

....

EMOTIONS/THOUGHTS: *How did you feel today?*

....

....

....

CONCERNS LIST: *What bothered you most today?*

....

....

....

GRATITUDE LIST: *What are you most grateful for today?*

....

....

....

DATE .... **YEAR** ....

FOOD: *What did you eat today?*

BREAKFAST: ....

Snack: ....

LUNCH: ....

Snack: ....

DINNER: ....

Snack: ....

DRINK: *What did you drink today?*

Any caffeinated drinks: ....

Any alcoholic drinks: ....

Any other drinks: ....

Any other drugs ingested: (including prescription, recreational, over the counter and nicotine) ....

....

QUICK CHECKLIST

WATER - how many litres? ⬚   MEDITATION - how many minutes? ⬚

SLEEP - how many hours? ⬚   EXERCISE - how many minutes? ⬚

LIFE EVENTS: *What happened today?*

....

....

....

EMOTIONS/THOUGHTS: *How did you feel today?*

....

....

....

CONCERNS LIST: *What bothered you most today?*

....

....

....

GRATITUDE LIST: *What are you most grateful for today?*

....

....

....

DATE .... **YEAR** ....

FOOD: *What did you eat today?*

BREAKFAST: ....

Snack: ....

LUNCH: ....

Snack: ....

DINNER: ....

Snack: ....

DRINK: *What did you drink today?*

Any caffeinated drinks: ....

Any alcoholic drinks: ....

Any other drinks: ....

Any other drugs ingested: (including prescription, recreational, over the counter and nicotine) ....

....

QUICK CHECKLIST

WATER - how many litres? ▨   MEDITATION - how many minutes? ▨

SLEEP - how many hours? ▨   EXERCISE - how many minutes? ▨

LIFE EVENTS: *What happened today?*

....

....

....

EMOTIONS/THOUGHTS: *How did you feel today?*

....

....

....

CONCERNS LIST: *What bothered you most today?*

....

....

....

GRATITUDE LIST: *What are you most grateful for today?*

....

....

....

DATE .... **YEAR** ....

FOOD: *What did you eat today?*

BREAKFAST: ....

Snack: ....

LUNCH: ....

Snack: ....

DINNER: ....

Snack: ....

DRINK: *What did you drink today?*

Any caffeinated drinks: ....

Any alcoholic drinks: ....

Any other drinks: ....

Any other drugs ingested: (including prescription, recreational, over the counter and nicotine) ....

....

QUICK CHECKLIST

WATER - how many litres? ☐   MEDITATION - how many minutes? ☐

SLEEP - how many hours? ☐   EXERCISE - how many minutes? ☐

LIFE EVENTS: *What happened today?*

....

....

....

EMOTIONS/THOUGHTS: *How did you feel today?*

....

....

....

CONCERNS LIST: *What bothered you most today?*

....

....

....

GRATITUDE LIST: *What are you most grateful for today?*

....

....

....

DATE .... **YEAR** ....

FOOD: *What did you eat today?*

BREAKFAST: ....

Snack: ....

LUNCH: ....

Snack: ....

DINNER: ....

Snack: ....

DRINK: *What did you drink today?*

Any caffeinated drinks: ....

Any alcoholic drinks: ....

Any other drinks: ....

Any other drugs ingested: (including prescription, recreational, over the counter and nicotine) ....

....

QUICK CHECKLIST

WATER - how many litres? ☐   MEDITATION - how many minutes? ☐

SLEEP - how many hours? ☐   EXERCISE - how many minutes? ☐

LIFE EVENTS: *What happened today?*

....

....

....

EMOTIONS/THOUGHTS: *How did you feel today?*

....

....

....

CONCERNS LIST: *What bothered you most today?*

....

....

....

GRATITUDE LIST: *What are you most grateful for today?*

....

....

....

DATE .... **YEAR** ....

FOOD: *What did you eat today?*

BREAKFAST: ....

Snack: ....

LUNCH: ....

Snack: ....

DINNER: ....

Snack: ....

DRINK: *What did you drink today?*

Any caffeinated drinks: ....

Any alcoholic drinks: ....

Any other drinks: ....

Any other drugs ingested: (including prescription, recreational, over the counter and nicotine) ....

....

QUICK CHECKLIST

WATER - how many litres?   MEDITATION - how many minutes?

SLEEP - how many hours?   EXERCISE - how many minutes?

LIFE EVENTS: *What happened today?*

....

....

....

EMOTIONS/THOUGHTS: *How did you feel today?*

....

....

....

CONCERNS LIST: *What bothered you most today?*

....

....

....

GRATITUDE LIST: *What are you most grateful for today?*

....

....

....

DATE .... **YEAR** ....

FOOD: *What did you eat today?*

BREAKFAST: ....

Snack: ....

LUNCH: ....

Snack: ....

DINNER: ....

Snack: ....

DRINK: *What did you drink today?*

Any caffeinated drinks: ....

Any alcoholic drinks: ....

Any other drinks: ....

Any other drugs ingested: (including prescription, recreational, over the counter and nicotine) ....

....

QUICK CHECKLIST

WATER - how many litres? ▨   MEDITATION - how many minutes? ▨

SLEEP - how many hours? ▨   EXERCISE - how many minutes? ▨

LIFE EVENTS: *What happened today?*

....

....

....

EMOTIONS/THOUGHTS: *How did you feel today?*

....

....

....

CONCERNS LIST: *What bothered you most today?*

....

....

....

GRATITUDE LIST: *What are you most grateful for today?*

....

....

....

DATE .... **YEAR** ....

FOOD: *What did you eat today?*

BREAKFAST: ....

Snack: ....

LUNCH: ....

Snack: ....

DINNER: ....

Snack: ....

DRINK: *What did you drink today?*

Any caffeinated drinks: ....

Any alcoholic drinks: ....

Any other drinks: ....

Any other drugs ingested: (including prescription, recreational, over the counter and nicotine) ....

....

QUICK CHECKLIST

WATER - how many litres? ☐   MEDITATION - how many minutes? ☐

SLEEP - how many hours? ☐   EXERCISE - how many minutes? ☐

LIFE EVENTS: *What happened today?*

....

....

....

EMOTIONS/THOUGHTS: *How did you feel today?*

....

....

....

CONCERNS LIST: *What bothered you most today?*

....

....

....

GRATITUDE LIST: *What are you most grateful for today?*

....

....

....

DATE .... **YEAR** ....

FOOD: *What did you eat today?*

BREAKFAST: ....

Snack: ....

LUNCH: ....

Snack: ....

DINNER: ....

Snack: ....

DRINK: *What did you drink today?*

Any caffeinated drinks: ....

Any alcoholic drinks: ....

Any other drinks: ....

Any other drugs ingested: (including prescription, recreational, over the counter and nicotine) ....

....

QUICK CHECKLIST

WATER - how many litres? ▨   MEDITATION - how many minutes? ▨

SLEEP - how many hours? ▨   EXERCISE - how many minutes? ▨

LIFE EVENTS: *What happened today?*

....

....

....

EMOTIONS/THOUGHTS: *How did you feel today?*

....

....

....

CONCERNS LIST: *What bothered you most today?*

....

....

....

GRATITUDE LIST: *What are you most grateful for today?*

....

....

....

DATE .... **YEAR** ....

FOOD: *What did you eat today?*

BREAKFAST: ....

Snack: ....

LUNCH: ....

Snack: ....

DINNER: ....

Snack: ....

DRINK: *What did you drink today?*

Any caffeinated drinks: ....

Any alcoholic drinks: ....

Any other drinks: ....

Any other drugs ingested: (including prescription, recreational, over the counter and nicotine) ....
....

QUICK CHECKLIST

WATER - how many litres? ▢   MEDITATION - how many minutes? ▢

SLEEP - how many hours? ▢   EXERCISE - how many minutes? ▢

LIFE EVENTS: *What happened today?*

....

....

....

EMOTIONS/THOUGHTS: *How did you feel today?*

....

....

....

CONCERNS LIST: *What bothered you most today?*

....

....

....

GRATITUDE LIST: *What are you most grateful for today?*

....

....

....

DATE .... **YEAR** ....

FOOD: *What did you eat today?*

BREAKFAST: ....

Snack: ....

LUNCH: ....

Snack: ....

DINNER: ....

Snack: ....

DRINK: *What did you drink today?*

Any caffeinated drinks: ....

Any alcoholic drinks: ....

Any other drinks: ....

Any other drugs ingested: (including prescription, recreational, over the counter and nicotine) ....
....

QUICK CHECKLIST

WATER - how many litres? ⬜   MEDITATION - how many minutes? ⬜

SLEEP - how many hours? ⬜   EXERCISE - how many minutes? ⬜

LIFE EVENTS: *What happened today?*

....

....

....

EMOTIONS/THOUGHTS: *How did you feel today?*

....

....

....

CONCERNS LIST: *What bothered you most today?*

....

....

....

GRATITUDE LIST: *What are you most grateful for today?*

....

....

....

DATE .... **YEAR** ....

FOOD: *What did you eat today?*

BREAKFAST: ....

Snack: ....

LUNCH: ....

Snack: ....

DINNER: ....

Snack: ....

DRINK: *What did you drink today?*

Any caffeinated drinks: ....

Any alcoholic drinks: ....

Any other drinks: ....

Any other drugs ingested: (including prescription, recreational, over the counter and nicotine) ....

QUICK CHECKLIST

WATER - how many litres? ☐   MEDITATION - how many minutes? ☐

SLEEP - how many hours? ☐   EXERCISE - how many minutes? ☐

LIFE EVENTS: *What happened today?*

....

....

....

EMOTIONS/THOUGHTS: *How did you feel today?*

....

....

....

CONCERNS LIST: *What bothered you most today?*

....

....

....

GRATITUDE LIST: *What are you most grateful for today?*

....

....

....

DATE .... **YEAR** ....

FOOD: *What did you eat today?*

BREAKFAST: ....

Snack: ....

LUNCH: ....

Snack: ....

DINNER: ....

Snack: ....

DRINK: *What did you drink today?*

Any caffeinated drinks: ....

Any alcoholic drinks: ....

Any other drinks: ....

Any other drugs ingested: (including prescription, recreational, over the counter and nicotine) ....

....

QUICK CHECKLIST

WATER - how many litres? ☐ MEDITATION - how many minutes? ☐

SLEEP - how many hours? ☐ EXERCISE - how many minutes? ☐

LIFE EVENTS: *What happened today?*

....

....

....

EMOTIONS/THOUGHTS: *How did you feel today?*

....

....

....

CONCERNS LIST: *What bothered you most today?*

....

....

....

GRATITUDE LIST: *What are you most grateful for today?*

....

....

....

DATE .... **YEAR** ....

FOOD: *What did you eat today?*

BREAKFAST: ....

Snack: ....

LUNCH: ....

Snack: ....

DINNER: ....

Snack: ....

DRINK: *What did you drink today?*

Any caffeinated drinks: ....

Any alcoholic drinks: ....

Any other drinks: ....

Any other drugs ingested: (including prescription, recreational, over the counter and nicotine) ....

....

QUICK CHECKLIST

WATER - how many litres? ▨   MEDITATION - how many minutes? ▨

SLEEP - how many hours? ▨   EXERCISE - how many minutes? ▨

LIFE EVENTS: *What happened today?*

....

....

....

EMOTIONS/THOUGHTS: *How did you feel today?*

....

....

....

CONCERNS LIST: *What bothered you most today?*

....

....

....

GRATITUDE LIST: *What are you most grateful for today?*

....

....

....

DATE .... **YEAR** ....

FOOD: *What did you eat today?*

BREAKFAST: ....

Snack: ....

LUNCH: ....

Snack: ....

DINNER: ....

Snack: ....

DRINK: *What did you drink today?*

Any caffeinated drinks: ....

Any alcoholic drinks: ....

Any other drinks: ....

Any other drugs ingested: (including prescription, recreational, over the counter and nicotine) ....

....

QUICK CHECKLIST

WATER - how many litres?   ▨   MEDITATION - how many minutes?   ▨

SLEEP - how many hours?   ▨   EXERCISE - how many minutes?   ▨

LIFE EVENTS: *What happened today?*

....

....

....

EMOTIONS/THOUGHTS: *How did you feel today?*

....

....

....

CONCERNS LIST: *What bothered you most today?*

....

....

....

GRATITUDE LIST: *What are you most grateful for today?*

....

....

....

DATE .... **YEAR** ....

FOOD: *What did you eat today?*

BREAKFAST: ....

Snack: ....

LUNCH: ....

Snack: ....

DINNER: ....

Snack: ....

DRINK: *What did you drink today?*

Any caffeinated drinks: ....

Any alcoholic drinks: ....

Any other drinks: ....

Any other drugs ingested: (including prescription, recreational, over the counter and nicotine) ....

....

QUICK CHECKLIST

WATER - how many litres? ⬜   MEDITATION - how many minutes? ⬜

SLEEP - how many hours? ⬜   EXERCISE - how many minutes? ⬜

LIFE EVENTS: *What happened today?*

....

....

....

EMOTIONS/THOUGHTS: *How did you feel today?*

....

....

....

CONCERNS LIST: *What bothered you most today?*

....

....

....

GRATITUDE LIST: *What are you most grateful for today?*

....

....

....

MONTH

TEN

<u>willpower, decision making and forming habits</u>

There is a theory that willpower is both finite and renewable, meaning that, like energy, you wake up in the morning with a certain amount and you use it up at a variable rate as you go through the day.

So, depending on how you spend your day, what your thought patterns are and the sort of decisions you make, you might only make it until mid-morning some days before you have used up all of your stores of willpower and given in to temptation. Or alternatively, if you're prepared and measured and you take good loving care of yourself, you'll be able to get through the day without getting derailed.

The trick is to make good, considered decisions; even the little ones that we might think are inconsequential. We need to appreciate that taking on too many things in any given day will drain our precious reserves and leave us depleted and vulnerable to temptation. It's at those times, when we feel drained, that we often reach for the old familiar thing, or the easiest thing, or the nearest thing - rather than the best thing.

I can't tell you how many times in the past I reached for a drink, a doughnut or a douchebag - when what I actually needed was a nap, or a bubble bath or a good book.

A habit is just a decision made over and over again, and can be broken down into three parts:
• the cue
• the behaviour
• and the reward

When we do something repetitively over a period of time, a habit is formed and it can feel automatic; as though we have no control over it, but we *do* have control over it and we can learn to apply that self-control. We absolutely can. Furthermore, habits can be broken and new, healthier habits can be learned in their place instead. You just need to put the right thought and effort in, but you can do it, and the first step is just believing that you can do it.

MONTH .... YEAR ....

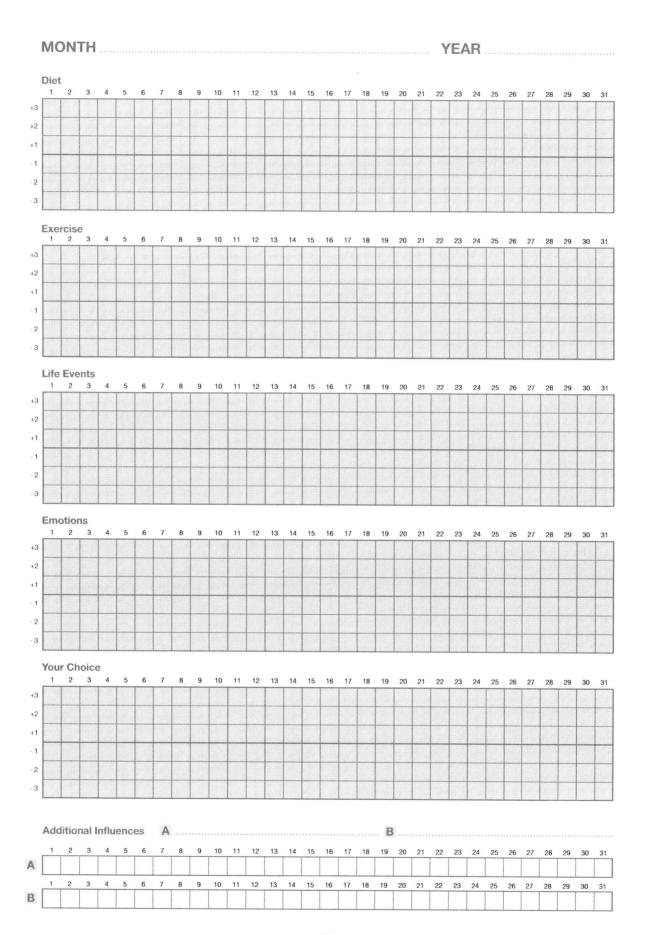

Diet

Exercise

Life Events

Emotions

Your Choice

Additional Influences   A ....   B ....

A

B

DATE .... **YEAR** ....

FOOD: *What did you eat today?*

BREAKFAST: ....

Snack: ....

LUNCH: ....

Snack: ....

DINNER: ....

Snack: ....

DRINK: *What did you drink today?*

Any caffeinated drinks: ....

Any alcoholic drinks: ....

Any other drinks: ....

Any other drugs ingested: (including prescription, recreational, over the counter and nicotine) ....

....

QUICK CHECKLIST

WATER - how many litres? ▢   MEDITATION - how many minutes? ▢

SLEEP - how many hours? ▢   EXERCISE - how many minutes? ▢

LIFE EVENTS: *What happened today?*

....

....

....

EMOTIONS/THOUGHTS: *How did you feel today?*

....

....

....

CONCERNS LIST: *What bothered you most today?*

....

....

....

GRATITUDE LIST: *What are you most grateful for today?*

....

....

....

DATE .... **YEAR** ....

FOOD: *What did you eat today?*

BREAKFAST: ....

Snack: ....

LUNCH: ....

Snack: ....

DINNER: ....

Snack: ....

DRINK: *What did you drink today?*

Any caffeinated drinks: ....

Any alcoholic drinks: ....

Any other drinks: ....

Any other drugs ingested: (including prescription, recreational, over the counter and nicotine) ....

....

QUICK CHECKLIST

WATER - how many litres? ☐   MEDITATION - how many minutes? ☐

SLEEP - how many hours? ☐   EXERCISE - how many minutes? ☐

LIFE EVENTS: *What happened today?*

....

....

....

EMOTIONS/THOUGHTS: *How did you feel today?*

....

....

....

CONCERNS LIST: *What bothered you most today?*

....

....

....

GRATITUDE LIST: *What are you most grateful for today?*

....

....

....

DATE .... **YEAR** ....

FOOD: *What did you eat today?*

BREAKFAST: ....

Snack: ....

LUNCH: ....

Snack: ....

DINNER: ....

Snack: ....

DRINK: *What did you drink today?*

Any caffeinated drinks: ....

Any alcoholic drinks: ....

Any other drinks: ....

Any other drugs ingested: (including prescription, recreational, over the counter and nicotine) ....
....

QUICK CHECKLIST

WATER - how many litres? ▫   MEDITATION - how many minutes? ▫

SLEEP - how many hours? ▫   EXERCISE - how many minutes? ▫

LIFE EVENTS: *What happened today?*

....
....
....

EMOTIONS/THOUGHTS: *How did you feel today?*

....
....
....

CONCERNS LIST: *What bothered you most today?*

....
....
....

GRATITUDE LIST: *What are you most grateful for today?*

....
....
....

DATE .... **YEAR** ....

FOOD: *What did you eat today?*

BREAKFAST: ....

Snack: ....

LUNCH: ....

Snack: ....

DINNER: ....

Snack: ....

DRINK: *What did you drink today?*

Any caffeinated drinks: ....

Any alcoholic drinks: ....

Any other drinks: ....

Any other drugs ingested: (including prescription, recreational, over the counter and nicotine) ....

....

QUICK CHECKLIST

WATER - how many litres? ☐   MEDITATION - how many minutes? ☐

SLEEP - how many hours? ☐   EXERCISE - how many minutes? ☐

LIFE EVENTS: *What happened today?*

....

....

....

EMOTIONS/THOUGHTS: *How did you feel today?*

....

....

....

CONCERNS LIST: *What bothered you most today?*

....

....

....

GRATITUDE LIST: *What are you most grateful for today?*

....

....

....

DATE .... **YEAR** ....

FOOD: *What did you eat today?*

BREAKFAST: ....

Snack: ....

LUNCH: ....

Snack: ....

DINNER: ....

Snack: ....

DRINK: *What did you drink today?*

Any caffeinated drinks: ....

Any alcoholic drinks: ....

Any other drinks: ....

Any other drugs ingested: (including prescription, recreational, over the counter and nicotine) ....

....

QUICK CHECKLIST

WATER - how many litres? ☐   MEDITATION - how many minutes? ☐

SLEEP - how many hours? ☐   EXERCISE - how many minutes? ☐

LIFE EVENTS: *What happened today?*

....

....

....

EMOTIONS/THOUGHTS: *How did you feel today?*

....

....

....

CONCERNS LIST: *What bothered you most today?*

....

....

....

GRATITUDE LIST: *What are you most grateful for today?*

....

....

....

DATE .... **YEAR** ....

FOOD: *What did you eat today?*

BREAKFAST: ....

Snack: ....

LUNCH: ....

Snack: ....

DINNER: ....

Snack: ....

DRINK: *What did you drink today?*

Any caffeinated drinks: ....

Any alcoholic drinks: ....

Any other drinks: ....

Any other drugs ingested: (including prescription, recreational, over the counter and nicotine) ....

....

QUICK CHECKLIST

WATER - how many litres? ▨   MEDITATION - how many minutes? ▨

SLEEP - how many hours? ▨   EXERCISE - how many minutes? ▨

LIFE EVENTS: *What happened today?*

....

....

....

EMOTIONS/THOUGHTS: *How did you feel today?*

....

....

....

CONCERNS LIST: *What bothered you most today?*

....

....

....

GRATITUDE LIST: *What are you most grateful for today?*

....

....

....

DATE .... **YEAR** ....

FOOD: *What did you eat today?*

BREAKFAST: ....

Snack: ....

LUNCH: ....

Snack: ....

DINNER: ....

Snack: ....

DRINK: *What did you drink today?*

Any caffeinated drinks: ....

Any alcoholic drinks: ....

Any other drinks: ....

Any other drugs ingested: (including prescription, recreational, over the counter and nicotine) ....

....

QUICK CHECKLIST

WATER - how many litres? ☐   MEDITATION - how many minutes? ☐

SLEEP - how many hours? ☐   EXERCISE - how many minutes? ☐

LIFE EVENTS: *What happened today?*

....

....

....

EMOTIONS/THOUGHTS: *How did you feel today?*

....

....

....

CONCERNS LIST: *What bothered you most today?*

....

....

....

GRATITUDE LIST: *What are you most grateful for today?*

....

....

....

DATE .... **YEAR** ....

FOOD: *What did you eat today?*

BREAKFAST: ....

Snack: ....

LUNCH: ....

Snack: ....

DINNER: ....

Snack: ....

DRINK: *What did you drink today?*

Any caffeinated drinks: ....

Any alcoholic drinks: ....

Any other drinks: ....

Any other drugs ingested: (including prescription, recreational, over the counter and nicotine) ....

....

QUICK CHECKLIST

WATER - how many litres? ☐   MEDITATION - how many minutes? ☐

SLEEP - how many hours? ☐   EXERCISE - how many minutes? ☐

LIFE EVENTS: *What happened today?*

....

....

....

EMOTIONS/THOUGHTS: *How did you feel today?*

....

....

....

CONCERNS LIST: *What bothered you most today?*

....

....

....

GRATITUDE LIST: *What are you most grateful for today?*

....

....

....

DATE .... **YEAR** ....

FOOD: *What did you eat today?*

BREAKFAST: ....

Snack: ....

LUNCH: ....

Snack: ....

DINNER: ....

Snack: ....

DRINK: *What did you drink today?*

Any caffeinated drinks: ....

Any alcoholic drinks: ....

Any other drinks: ....

Any other drugs ingested: (including prescription, recreational, over the counter and nicotine) ....

....

QUICK CHECKLIST

WATER - how many litres? ☐   MEDITATION - how many minutes? ☐

SLEEP - how many hours? ☐   EXERCISE - how many minutes? ☐

LIFE EVENTS: *What happened today?*

....

....

....

EMOTIONS/THOUGHTS: *How did you feel today?*

....

....

....

CONCERNS LIST: *What bothered you most today?*

....

....

....

GRATITUDE LIST: *What are you most grateful for today?*

....

....

....

DATE .... **YEAR** ....

FOOD: *What did you eat today?*

BREAKFAST: ....

Snack: ....

LUNCH: ....

Snack: ....

DINNER: ....

Snack: ....

DRINK: *What did you drink today?*

Any caffeinated drinks: ....

Any alcoholic drinks: ....

Any other drinks: ....

Any other drugs ingested: (including prescription, recreational, over the counter and nicotine) ....

....

QUICK CHECKLIST

WATER - how many litres? ☐   MEDITATION - how many minutes? ☐

SLEEP - how many hours? ☐   EXERCISE - how many minutes? ☐

LIFE EVENTS: *What happened today?*

....

....

....

EMOTIONS/THOUGHTS: *How did you feel today?*

....

....

....

CONCERNS LIST: *What bothered you most today?*

....

....

....

GRATITUDE LIST: *What are you most grateful for today?*

....

....

....

DATE .... **YEAR** ....

FOOD: *What did you eat today?*

BREAKFAST: ....

Snack: ....

LUNCH: ....

Snack: ....

DINNER: ....

Snack: ....

DRINK: *What did you drink today?*

Any caffeinated drinks: ....

Any alcoholic drinks: ....

Any other drinks: ....

Any other drugs ingested: (including prescription, recreational, over the counter and nicotine) ....

....

QUICK CHECKLIST

WATER - how many litres? ☐   MEDITATION - how many minutes? ☐

SLEEP - how many hours? ☐   EXERCISE - how many minutes? ☐

LIFE EVENTS: *What happened today?*

....

....

....

EMOTIONS/THOUGHTS: *How did you feel today?*

....

....

....

CONCERNS LIST: *What bothered you most today?*

....

....

....

GRATITUDE LIST: *What are you most grateful for today?*

....

....

....

DATE .... **YEAR** ....

FOOD: *What did you eat today?*

BREAKFAST: ....

Snack: ....

LUNCH: ....

Snack: ....

DINNER: ....

Snack: ....

DRINK: *What did you drink today?*

Any caffeinated drinks: ....

Any alcoholic drinks: ....

Any other drinks: ....

Any other drugs ingested: (including prescription, recreational, over the counter and nicotine) ....

....

QUICK CHECKLIST

WATER - how many litres? ☐   MEDITATION - how many minutes? ☐

SLEEP - how many hours? ☐   EXERCISE - how many minutes? ☐

LIFE EVENTS: *What happened today?*

....

....

....

EMOTIONS/THOUGHTS: *How did you feel today?*

....

....

....

CONCERNS LIST: *What bothered you most today?*

....

....

....

GRATITUDE LIST: *What are you most grateful for today?*

....

....

....

DATE .... **YEAR** ....

FOOD: *What did you eat today?*

BREAKFAST: ....

Snack: ....

LUNCH: ....

Snack: ....

DINNER: ....

Snack: ....

DRINK: *What did you drink today?*

Any caffeinated drinks: ....

Any alcoholic drinks: ....

Any other drinks: ....

Any other drugs ingested: (including prescription, recreational, over the counter and nicotine) ....

....

QUICK CHECKLIST

WATER - how many litres? ☐   MEDITATION - how many minutes? ☐

SLEEP - how many hours? ☐   EXERCISE - how many minutes? ☐

LIFE EVENTS: *What happened today?*

....

....

....

EMOTIONS/THOUGHTS: *How did you feel today?*

....

....

....

CONCERNS LIST: *What bothered you most today?*

....

....

....

GRATITUDE LIST: *What are you most grateful for today?*

....

....

....

DATE .... **YEAR** ....

FOOD: *What did you eat today?*

BREAKFAST: ....

Snack: ....

LUNCH: ....

Snack: ....

DINNER: ....

Snack: ....

DRINK: *What did you drink today?*

Any caffeinated drinks: ....

Any alcoholic drinks: ....

Any other drinks: ....

Any other drugs ingested: (including prescription, recreational, over the counter and nicotine) ....

....

QUICK CHECKLIST

WATER - how many litres? ▢   MEDITATION - how many minutes? ▢

SLEEP - how many hours? ▢   EXERCISE - how many minutes? ▢

LIFE EVENTS: *What happened today?*

....

....

....

EMOTIONS/THOUGHTS: *How did you feel today?*

....

....

....

CONCERNS LIST: *What bothered you most today?*

....

....

....

GRATITUDE LIST: *What are you most grateful for today?*

....

....

....

DATE .... **YEAR** ....

FOOD: *What did you eat today?*

BREAKFAST: ....

Snack: ....

LUNCH: ....

Snack: ....

DINNER: ....

Snack: ....

DRINK: *What did you drink today?*

Any caffeinated drinks: ....

Any alcoholic drinks: ....

Any other drinks: ....

Any other drugs ingested: (including prescription, recreational, over the counter and nicotine) ....

....

QUICK CHECKLIST

WATER - how many litres? ▢   MEDITATION - how many minutes? ▢

SLEEP - how many hours? ▢   EXERCISE - how many minutes? ▢

LIFE EVENTS: *What happened today?*

....

....

....

EMOTIONS/THOUGHTS: *How did you feel today?*

....

....

....

CONCERNS LIST: *What bothered you most today?*

....

....

....

GRATITUDE LIST: *What are you most grateful for today?*

....

....

....

DATE .... **YEAR** ....

FOOD: *What did you eat today?*

BREAKFAST: ....

Snack: ....

LUNCH: ....

Snack: ....

DINNER: ....

Snack: ....

DRINK: *What did you drink today?*

Any caffeinated drinks: ....

Any alcoholic drinks: ....

Any other drinks: ....

Any other drugs ingested: (including prescription, recreational, over the counter and nicotine) ....

....

QUICK CHECKLIST

WATER - how many litres? ☐   MEDITATION - how many minutes? ☐

SLEEP - how many hours? ☐   EXERCISE - how many minutes? ☐

LIFE EVENTS: *What happened today?*

....

....

....

EMOTIONS/THOUGHTS: *How did you feel today?*

....

....

....

CONCERNS LIST: *What bothered you most today?*

....

....

....

GRATITUDE LIST: *What are you most grateful for today?*

....

....

....

DATE .... **YEAR** ....

FOOD: *What did you eat today?*

BREAKFAST: ....

Snack: ....

LUNCH: ....

Snack: ....

DINNER: ....

Snack: ....

DRINK: *What did you drink today?*

Any caffeinated drinks: ....

Any alcoholic drinks: ....

Any other drinks: ....

Any other drugs ingested: (including prescription, recreational, over the counter and nicotine) ....

....

QUICK CHECKLIST

WATER - how many litres? ☐   MEDITATION - how many minutes? ☐

SLEEP - how many hours? ☐   EXERCISE - how many minutes? ☐

LIFE EVENTS: *What happened today?*

....

....

....

EMOTIONS/THOUGHTS: *How did you feel today?*

....

....

....

CONCERNS LIST: *What bothered you most today?*

....

....

....

GRATITUDE LIST: *What are you most grateful for today?*

....

....

....

DATE .... **YEAR** ....

FOOD: *What did you eat today?*

BREAKFAST: ....

Snack: ....

LUNCH: ....

Snack: ....

DINNER: ....

Snack: ....

DRINK: *What did you drink today?*

Any caffeinated drinks: ....

Any alcoholic drinks: ....

Any other drinks: ....

Any other drugs ingested: (including prescription, recreational, over the counter and nicotine) ....

....

QUICK CHECKLIST

WATER - how many litres? ▨   MEDITATION - how many minutes? ▨

SLEEP - how many hours? ▨   EXERCISE - how many minutes? ▨

LIFE EVENTS: *What happened today?*

....

....

....

EMOTIONS/THOUGHTS: *How did you feel today?*

....

....

....

CONCERNS LIST: *What bothered you most today?*

....

....

....

GRATITUDE LIST: *What are you most grateful for today?*

....

....

....

DATE .... **YEAR** ....

FOOD: *What did you eat today?*

BREAKFAST: ....

Snack: ....

LUNCH: ....

Snack: ....

DINNER: ....

Snack: ....

DRINK: *What did you drink today?*

Any caffeinated drinks: ....

Any alcoholic drinks: ....

Any other drinks: ....

Any other drugs ingested: (including prescription, recreational, over the counter and nicotine) ....

....

QUICK CHECKLIST

WATER - how many litres? ☐   MEDITATION - how many minutes? ☐

SLEEP - how many hours? ☐   EXERCISE - how many minutes? ☐

LIFE EVENTS: *What happened today?*

....

....

....

EMOTIONS/THOUGHTS: *How did you feel today?*

....

....

....

CONCERNS LIST: *What bothered you most today?*

....

....

....

GRATITUDE LIST: *What are you most grateful for today?*

....

....

....

DATE .... **YEAR** ....

FOOD: *What did you eat today?*

BREAKFAST: ....

Snack: ....

LUNCH: ....

Snack: ....

DINNER: ....

Snack: ....

DRINK: *What did you drink today?*

Any caffeinated drinks: ....

Any alcoholic drinks: ....

Any other drinks: ....

Any other drugs ingested: (including prescription, recreational, over the counter and nicotine) ....

....

QUICK CHECKLIST

WATER - how many litres? ☐ MEDITATION - how many minutes? ☐

SLEEP - how many hours? ☐ EXERCISE - how many minutes? ☐

LIFE EVENTS: *What happened today?*

....

....

....

EMOTIONS/THOUGHTS: *How did you feel today?*

....

....

....

CONCERNS LIST: *What bothered you most today?*

....

....

....

GRATITUDE LIST: *What are you most grateful for today?*

....

....

....

DATE .... **YEAR** ....

FOOD: *What did you eat today?*

BREAKFAST: ....

Snack: ....

LUNCH: ....

Snack: ....

DINNER: ....

Snack: ....

DRINK: *What did you drink today?*

Any caffeinated drinks: ....

Any alcoholic drinks: ....

Any other drinks: ....

Any other drugs ingested: (including prescription, recreational, over the counter and nicotine) ....

....

QUICK CHECKLIST

WATER - how many litres? ☐   MEDITATION - how many minutes? ☐

SLEEP - how many hours? ☐   EXERCISE - how many minutes? ☐

LIFE EVENTS: *What happened today?*

....

....

....

EMOTIONS/THOUGHTS: *How did you feel today?*

....

....

....

CONCERNS LIST: *What bothered you most today?*

....

....

....

GRATITUDE LIST: *What are you most grateful for today?*

....

....

....

DATE .... **YEAR** ....

FOOD: *What did you eat today?*

BREAKFAST: ....

Snack: ....

LUNCH: ....

Snack: ....

DINNER: ....

Snack: ....

DRINK: *What did you drink today?*

Any caffeinated drinks: ....

Any alcoholic drinks: ....

Any other drinks: ....

Any other drugs ingested: (including prescription, recreational, over the counter and nicotine) ....

....

QUICK CHECKLIST

WATER - how many litres? ☐   MEDITATION - how many minutes? ☐

SLEEP - how many hours? ☐   EXERCISE - how many minutes? ☐

LIFE EVENTS: *What happened today?*

....

....

....

EMOTIONS/THOUGHTS: *How did you feel today?*

....

....

....

CONCERNS LIST: *What bothered you most today?*

....

....

....

GRATITUDE LIST: *What are you most grateful for today?*

....

....

....

DATE .... **YEAR** ....

FOOD: *What did you eat today?*

BREAKFAST: ....

Snack: ....

LUNCH: ....

Snack: ....

DINNER: ....

Snack: ....

DRINK: *What did you drink today?*

Any caffeinated drinks: ....

Any alcoholic drinks: ....

Any other drinks: ....

Any other drugs ingested: (including prescription, recreational, over the counter and nicotine) ....

....

QUICK CHECKLIST

WATER - how many litres? ☐   MEDITATION - how many minutes? ☐

SLEEP - how many hours? ☐   EXERCISE - how many minutes? ☐

LIFE EVENTS: *What happened today?*

....

....

....

EMOTIONS/THOUGHTS: *How did you feel today?*

....

....

....

CONCERNS LIST: *What bothered you most today?*

....

....

....

GRATITUDE LIST: *What are you most grateful for today?*

....

....

....

DATE .... **YEAR** ....

FOOD: *What did you eat today?*

BREAKFAST: ....

Snack: ....

LUNCH: ....

Snack: ....

DINNER: ....

Snack: ....

DRINK: *What did you drink today?*

Any caffeinated drinks: ....

Any alcoholic drinks: ....

Any other drinks: ....

Any other drugs ingested: (including prescription, recreational, over the counter and nicotine) ....

....

QUICK CHECKLIST

WATER - how many litres? ▨   MEDITATION - how many minutes? ▨

SLEEP - how many hours? ▨   EXERCISE - how many minutes? ▨

LIFE EVENTS: *What happened today?*

....

....

....

EMOTIONS/THOUGHTS: *How did you feel today?*

....

....

....

CONCERNS LIST: *What bothered you most today?*

....

....

....

GRATITUDE LIST: *What are you most grateful for today?*

....

....

....

DATE .... **YEAR** ....

FOOD: *What did you eat today?*

BREAKFAST: ....

Snack: ....

LUNCH: ....

Snack: ....

DINNER: ....

Snack: ....

DRINK: *What did you drink today?*

Any caffeinated drinks: ....

Any alcoholic drinks: ....

Any other drinks: ....

Any other drugs ingested: (including prescription, recreational, over the counter and nicotine) ....

....

QUICK CHECKLIST

WATER - how many litres? ▢   MEDITATION - how many minutes? ▢

SLEEP - how many hours? ▢   EXERCISE - how many minutes? ▢

LIFE EVENTS: *What happened today?*

....

....

....

EMOTIONS/THOUGHTS: *How did you feel today?*

....

....

....

CONCERNS LIST: *What bothered you most today?*

....

....

....

GRATITUDE LIST: *What are you most grateful for today?*

....

....

....

DATE .... **YEAR** ....

FOOD: *What did you eat today?*

BREAKFAST: ....

Snack: ....

LUNCH: ....

Snack: ....

DINNER: ....

Snack: ....

DRINK: *What did you drink today?*

Any caffeinated drinks: ....

Any alcoholic drinks: ....

Any other drinks: ....

Any other drugs ingested: (including prescription, recreational, over the counter and nicotine) ....

....

QUICK CHECKLIST

WATER - how many litres? ☐   MEDITATION - how many minutes? ☐

SLEEP - how many hours? ☐   EXERCISE - how many minutes? ☐

LIFE EVENTS: *What happened today?*

....

....

....

EMOTIONS/THOUGHTS: *How did you feel today?*

....

....

....

CONCERNS LIST: *What bothered you most today?*

....

....

....

GRATITUDE LIST: *What are you most grateful for today?*

....

....

....

DATE .... **YEAR** ....

FOOD: *What did you eat today?*

BREAKFAST: ....

Snack: ....

LUNCH: ....

Snack: ....

DINNER: ....

Snack: ....

DRINK: *What did you drink today?*

Any caffeinated drinks: ....

Any alcoholic drinks: ....

Any other drinks: ....

Any other drugs ingested: (including prescription, recreational, over the counter and nicotine) ....

....

QUICK CHECKLIST

WATER - how many litres? ☐   MEDITATION - how many minutes? ☐

SLEEP - how many hours? ☐   EXERCISE - how many minutes? ☐

LIFE EVENTS: *What happened today?*

....

....

....

EMOTIONS/THOUGHTS: *How did you feel today?*

....

....

....

CONCERNS LIST: *What bothered you most today?*

....

....

....

GRATITUDE LIST: *What are you most grateful for today?*

....

....

....

DATE .... **YEAR** ....

FOOD: *What did you eat today?*

BREAKFAST: ....

Snack: ....

LUNCH: ....

Snack: ....

DINNER: ....

Snack: ....

DRINK: *What did you drink today?*

Any caffeinated drinks: ....

Any alcoholic drinks: ....

Any other drinks: ....

Any other drugs ingested: (including prescription, recreational, over the counter and nicotine) ....

....

QUICK CHECKLIST

WATER - how many litres? ▨   MEDITATION - how many minutes? ▨

SLEEP - how many hours? ▨   EXERCISE - how many minutes? ▨

LIFE EVENTS: *What happened today?*

....

....

....

EMOTIONS/THOUGHTS: *How did you feel today?*

....

....

....

CONCERNS LIST: *What bothered you most today?*

....

....

....

GRATITUDE LIST: *What are you most grateful for today?*

....

....

....

DATE .... **YEAR** ....

FOOD: *What did you eat today?*

BREAKFAST: ....

Snack: ....

LUNCH: ....

Snack: ....

DINNER: ....

Snack: ....

DRINK: *What did you drink today?*

Any caffeinated drinks: ....

Any alcoholic drinks: ....

Any other drinks: ....

Any other drugs ingested: (including prescription, recreational, over the counter and nicotine) ....

....

QUICK CHECKLIST

WATER - how many litres? ▓   MEDITATION - how many minutes? ▓

SLEEP - how many hours? ▓   EXERCISE - how many minutes? ▓

LIFE EVENTS: *What happened today?*

....

....

....

EMOTIONS/THOUGHTS: *How did you feel today?*

....

....

....

CONCERNS LIST: *What bothered you most today?*

....

....

....

GRATITUDE LIST: *What are you most grateful for today?*

....

....

....

DATE .... **YEAR** ....

FOOD: *What did you eat today?*

BREAKFAST: ....

Snack: ....

LUNCH: ....

Snack: ....

DINNER: ....

Snack: ....

DRINK: *What did you drink today?*

Any caffeinated drinks: ....

Any alcoholic drinks: ....

Any other drinks: ....

Any other drugs ingested: (including prescription, recreational, over the counter and nicotine) ....

....

QUICK CHECKLIST

WATER - how many litres? ▨   MEDITATION - how many minutes? ▨

SLEEP - how many hours? ▨   EXERCISE - how many minutes? ▨

LIFE EVENTS: *What happened today?*

....

....

....

EMOTIONS/THOUGHTS: *How did you feel today?*

....

....

....

CONCERNS LIST: *What bothered you most today?*

....

....

....

GRATITUDE LIST: *What are you most grateful for today?*

....

....

....

DATE .... **YEAR** ....

FOOD: *What did you eat today?*

BREAKFAST: ....

Snack: ....

LUNCH: ....

Snack: ....

DINNER: ....

Snack: ....

DRINK: *What did you drink today?*

Any caffeinated drinks: ....

Any alcoholic drinks: ....

Any other drinks: ....

Any other drugs ingested: (including prescription, recreational, over the counter and nicotine) ....

....

QUICK CHECKLIST

WATER - how many litres? ☐   MEDITATION - how many minutes? ☐

SLEEP - how many hours? ☐   EXERCISE - how many minutes? ☐

LIFE EVENTS: *What happened today?*

....

....

....

EMOTIONS/THOUGHTS: *How did you feel today?*

....

....

....

CONCERNS LIST: *What bothered you most today?*

....

....

....

GRATITUDE LIST: *What are you most grateful for today?*

....

....

....

MONTH

ELEVEN

sleep and caffeine

Getting enough good quality kip every night is absolutely crucial to your physical and mental health. How well you function while you're awake is largely contingent on how well you sleep. When you're asleep, your body is working incredibly hard to heal, repair and rejuvenate itself. While you're sound asleep, dreaming, snoring, dribbling, whatever (no judgement here), a colossal amount of restoration work is taking place. Hormones are being balanced. Cells are being renewed. Brain function is revived. There is not a single part of your body that doesn't benefit from a nice deep sleep.

Conversely, when you're sleep deprived, you're buggered on an elemental level: You have difficulty making decisions and solving problems. You're emotionally unbalanced. You're erratic, forgetful and more physically fragile. You're clumsy and grumpy and snappy. We all know what a bad night's sleep does to us on a conscious level but the long-term negative effects are far-reaching and can become chronic. Sleep deprivation has strong links to depression, anxiety and hundreds of other health issues. Which, in turn is linked to people developing unhealthy coping strategies, with food, drink, drugs, other people and so on, instead of addressing the root cause of the problem.

For example, sleep deprivation is synonymous with caffeine dependency. We've all heard people making light of it: "don't talk to me until I've had my coffee" is a commonplace joke, but is it funny to be that reliant on anything? Caffeine is not a necessity, far from it, and yet so many people admit that they can't function on a basic everyday level without it. Caffeine is a commonplace, widespread drug, but that doesn't necessarily mean that it's good for us to consume it in such compulsive and copious ways. It is a strong, psychoactive, addictive stimulant that negatively affects and severely compromises the central nervous system. It acts in the human body as as adenosine receptor antagonist. Adenosine is the substance in the body that promotes sleep. Caffeine interferes with that system, raising your blood pressure, increasing your heart rate and inducing a state of being alert. It's a fast-acting drug that even in moderate doses can cause palpitations, tachycardia, digestive upset, sweating, nausea, insomnia, mania, irritability and induce feelings of high anxiety. If you're not enjoying the benefits of a good nights sleep, consider cutting down on the caffeine.

If you love the smell and the taste of caffeinated drinks, or want to wean off them gradually, trying switching to de-caff alternatives - all the flavour without the sleep-thieving qualities.

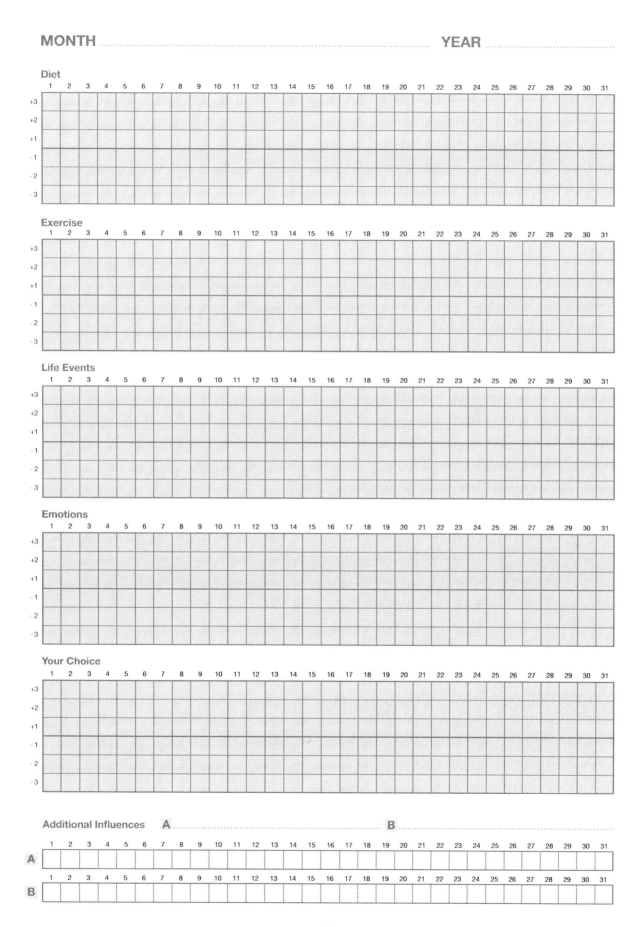

DATE .... **YEAR** ....

FOOD: *What did you eat today?*

BREAKFAST: ....

Snack: ....

LUNCH: ....

Snack: ....

DINNER: ....

Snack: ....

DRINK: *What did you drink today?*

Any caffeinated drinks: ....

Any alcoholic drinks: ....

Any other drinks: ....

Any other drugs ingested: (including prescription, recreational, over the counter and nicotine) ....

....

QUICK CHECKLIST

WATER - how many litres? ☐   MEDITATION - how many minutes? ☐

SLEEP - how many hours? ☐   EXERCISE - how many minutes? ☐

LIFE EVENTS: *What happened today?*

....

....

....

EMOTIONS/THOUGHTS: *How did you feel today?*

....

....

....

CONCERNS LIST: *What bothered you most today?*

....

....

....

GRATITUDE LIST: *What are you most grateful for today?*

....

....

....

DATE .... **YEAR** ....

FOOD: *What did you eat today?*

BREAKFAST: ....

Snack: ....

LUNCH: ....

Snack: ....

DINNER: ....

Snack: ....

DRINK: *What did you drink today?*

Any caffeinated drinks: ....

Any alcoholic drinks: ....

Any other drinks: ....

Any other drugs ingested: (including prescription, recreational, over the counter and nicotine) ....

....

QUICK CHECKLIST

WATER - how many litres? ▨   MEDITATION - how many minutes? ▨

SLEEP - how many hours? ▨   EXERCISE - how many minutes? ▨

LIFE EVENTS: *What happened today?*

....

....

....

EMOTIONS/THOUGHTS: *How did you feel today?*

....

....

....

CONCERNS LIST: *What bothered you most today?*

....

....

....

GRATITUDE LIST: *What are you most grateful for today?*

....

....

....

DATE .... **YEAR** ....

FOOD: *What did you eat today?*

BREAKFAST: ....

Snack: ....

LUNCH: ....

Snack: ....

DINNER: ....

Snack: ....

DRINK: *What did you drink today?*

Any caffeinated drinks: ....

Any alcoholic drinks: ....

Any other drinks: ....

Any other drugs ingested: (including prescription, recreational, over the counter and nicotine) ....

....

QUICK CHECKLIST

WATER - how many litres? ☐   MEDITATION - how many minutes? ☐

SLEEP - how many hours? ☐   EXERCISE - how many minutes? ☐

LIFE EVENTS: *What happened today?*

....

....

....

EMOTIONS/THOUGHTS: *How did you feel today?*

....

....

....

CONCERNS LIST: *What bothered you most today?*

....

....

....

GRATITUDE LIST: *What are you most grateful for today?*

....

....

....

DATE .... **YEAR** ....

FOOD: *What did you eat today?*

BREAKFAST: ....,........................

Snack: ....

LUNCH: ....

Snack: ....

DINNER: ....

Snack: ....

DRINK: *What did you drink today?*

Any caffeinated drinks: ....

Any alcoholic drinks: ....

Any other drinks: ....

Any other drugs ingested: (including prescription, recreational, over the counter and nicotine) ....

....

QUICK CHECKLIST

WATER - how many litres? ☐   MEDITATION - how many minutes? ☐

SLEEP - how many hours? ☐   EXERCISE - how many minutes? ☐

LIFE EVENTS: *What happened today?*

....

....

....

EMOTIONS/THOUGHTS: *How did you feel today?*

....

....

....

CONCERNS LIST: *What bothered you most today?*

....

....

....

GRATITUDE LIST: *What are you most grateful for today?*

....

....

....

DATE .... **YEAR** ....

FOOD: *What did you eat today?*

BREAKFAST: ....

Snack: ....

LUNCH: ....

Snack: ....

DINNER: ....

Snack: ....

DRINK: *What did you drink today?*

Any caffeinated drinks: ....

Any alcoholic drinks: ....

Any other drinks: ....

Any other drugs ingested: (including prescription, recreational, over the counter and nicotine) ....

....

QUICK CHECKLIST

WATER - how many litres? ☐   MEDITATION - how many minutes? ☐

SLEEP - how many hours? ☐   EXERCISE - how many minutes? ☐

LIFE EVENTS: *What happened today?*

....

....

....

EMOTIONS/THOUGHTS: *How did you feel today?*

....

....

....

CONCERNS LIST: *What bothered you most today?*

....

....

....

GRATITUDE LIST: *What are you most grateful for today?*

....

....

....

DATE .... **YEAR** ....

FOOD: *What did you eat today?*

BREAKFAST: ....

Snack: ....

LUNCH: ....

Snack: ....

DINNER: ....

Snack: ....

DRINK: *What did you drink today?*

Any caffeinated drinks: ....

Any alcoholic drinks: ....

Any other drinks: ....

Any other drugs ingested: (including prescription, recreational, over the counter and nicotine) ....

....

QUICK CHECKLIST

WATER - how many litres? ☐   MEDITATION - how many minutes? ☐

SLEEP - how many hours? ☐   EXERCISE - how many minutes? ☐

LIFE EVENTS: *What happened today?*

....

....

....

EMOTIONS/THOUGHTS: *How did you feel today?*

....

....

....

CONCERNS LIST: *What bothered you most today?*

....

....

....

GRATITUDE LIST: *What are you most grateful for today?*

....

....

....

DATE .... **YEAR** ....

FOOD: *What did you eat today?*

BREAKFAST: ....

Snack: ....

LUNCH: ....

Snack: ....

DINNER: ....

Snack: ....

DRINK: *What did you drink today?*

Any caffeinated drinks: ....

Any alcoholic drinks: ....

Any other drinks: ....

Any other drugs ingested: (including prescription, recreational, over the counter and nicotine) ....

....

QUICK CHECKLIST

WATER - how many litres? ☐   MEDITATION - how many minutes? ☐

SLEEP - how many hours? ☐   EXERCISE - how many minutes? ☐

LIFE EVENTS: *What happened today?*

....

....

....

EMOTIONS/THOUGHTS: *How did you feel today?*

....

....

....

CONCERNS LIST: *What bothered you most today?*

....

....

....

GRATITUDE LIST: *What are you most grateful for today?*

....

....

....

DATE .... **YEAR** ....

FOOD: *What did you eat today?*

BREAKFAST: ....

Snack: ....

LUNCH: ....

Snack: ....

DINNER: ....

Snack: ....

DRINK: *What did you drink today?*

Any caffeinated drinks: ....

Any alcoholic drinks: ....

Any other drinks: ....

Any other drugs ingested: (including prescription, recreational, over the counter and nicotine) ....

....

QUICK CHECKLIST

WATER - how many litres? ☐   MEDITATION - how many minutes? ☐

SLEEP - how many hours? ☐   EXERCISE - how many minutes? ☐

LIFE EVENTS: *What happened today?*

....

....

....

EMOTIONS/THOUGHTS: *How did you feel today?*

....

....

....

CONCERNS LIST: *What bothered you most today?*

....

....

....

GRATITUDE LIST: *What are you most grateful for today?*

....

....

....

DATE .... **YEAR** ....

FOOD: *What did you eat today?*

BREAKFAST: ....

Snack: ....

LUNCH: ....

Snack: ....

DINNER: ....

Snack: ....

DRINK: *What did you drink today?*

Any caffeinated drinks: ....

Any alcoholic drinks: ....

Any other drinks: ....

Any other drugs ingested: (including prescription, recreational, over the counter and nicotine) ....

....

QUICK CHECKLIST

WATER - how many litres? ▢   MEDITATION - how many minutes? ▢

SLEEP - how many hours? ▢   EXERCISE - how many minutes? ▢

LIFE EVENTS: *What happened today?*

....

....

....

EMOTIONS/THOUGHTS: *How did you feel today?*

....

....

....

CONCERNS LIST: *What bothered you most today?*

....

....

....

GRATITUDE LIST: *What are you most grateful for today?*

....

....

....

DATE .... **YEAR** ....

FOOD: *What did you eat today?*

BREAKFAST: ....

Snack: ....

LUNCH: ....

Snack: ....

DINNER: ....

Snack: ....

DRINK: *What did you drink today?*

Any caffeinated drinks: ....

Any alcoholic drinks: ....

Any other drinks: ....

Any other drugs ingested: (including prescription, recreational, over the counter and nicotine) ....

....

QUICK CHECKLIST

WATER - how many litres? ▢   MEDITATION - how many minutes? ▢

SLEEP - how many hours? ▢   EXERCISE - how many minutes? ▢

LIFE EVENTS: *What happened today?*

....

....

....

EMOTIONS/THOUGHTS: *How did you feel today?*

....

....

....

CONCERNS LIST: *What bothered you most today?*

....

....

....

GRATITUDE LIST: *What are you most grateful for today?*

....

....

....

DATE .... **YEAR** ....

FOOD: *What did you eat today?*

BREAKFAST: ....

Snack: ....

LUNCH: ....

Snack: ....

DINNER: ....

Snack: ....

DRINK: *What did you drink today?*

Any caffeinated drinks: ....

Any alcoholic drinks: ....

Any other drinks: ....

Any other drugs ingested: (including prescription, recreational, over the counter and nicotine) ....
....

QUICK CHECKLIST

WATER - how many litres? ▢   MEDITATION - how many minutes? ▢

SLEEP - how many hours? ▢   EXERCISE - how many minutes? ▢

LIFE EVENTS: *What happened today?*

....

....

....

EMOTIONS/THOUGHTS: *How did you feel today?*

....

....

....

CONCERNS LIST: *What bothered you most today?*

....

....

....

GRATITUDE LIST: *What are you most grateful for today?*

....

....

....

DATE .... **YEAR** ....

FOOD: *What did you eat today?*

BREAKFAST: ....

Snack: ....

LUNCH: ....

Snack: ....

DINNER: ....

Snack: ....

DRINK: *What did you drink today?*

Any caffeinated drinks: ....

Any alcoholic drinks: ....

Any other drinks: ....

Any other drugs ingested: (including prescription, recreational, over the counter and nicotine) ....

....

QUICK CHECKLIST

WATER - how many litres? ☐   MEDITATION - how many minutes? ☐

SLEEP - how many hours? ☐   EXERCISE - how many minutes? ☐

LIFE EVENTS: *What happened today?*

....

....

....

EMOTIONS/THOUGHTS: *How did you feel today?*

....

....

....

CONCERNS LIST: *What bothered you most today?*

....

....

....

GRATITUDE LIST: *What are you most grateful for today?*

....

....

....

DATE .... **YEAR** ....

FOOD: *What did you eat today?*

BREAKFAST: ....

Snack: ....

LUNCH: ....

Snack: ....

DINNER: ....

Snack: ....

DRINK: *What did you drink today?*

Any caffeinated drinks: ....

Any alcoholic drinks: ....

Any other drinks: ....

Any other drugs ingested: (including prescription, recreational, over the counter and nicotine) ....

....

QUICK CHECKLIST

WATER - how many litres? ☐   MEDITATION - how many minutes? ☐

SLEEP - how many hours? ☐   EXERCISE - how many minutes? ☐

LIFE EVENTS: *What happened today?*

....

....

....

EMOTIONS/THOUGHTS: *How did you feel today?*

....

....

....

CONCERNS LIST: *What bothered you most today?*

....

....

....

GRATITUDE LIST: *What are you most grateful for today?*

....

....

....

DATE .... **YEAR** ....

FOOD: *What did you eat today?*

BREAKFAST: ....

Snack: ....

LUNCH: ....

Snack: ....

DINNER: ....

Snack: ....

DRINK: *What did you drink today?*

Any caffeinated drinks: ....

Any alcoholic drinks: ....

Any other drinks: ....

Any other drugs ingested: (including prescription, recreational, over the counter and nicotine) ....

....

QUICK CHECKLIST

WATER - how many litres? ▨   MEDITATION - how many minutes? ▨

SLEEP - how many hours? ▨   EXERCISE - how many minutes? ▨

LIFE EVENTS: *What happened today?*

....

....

....

EMOTIONS/THOUGHTS: *How did you feel today?*

....

....

....

CONCERNS LIST: *What bothered you most today?*

....

....

....

GRATITUDE LIST: *What are you most grateful for today?*

....

....

....

DATE .... **YEAR** ....

FOOD: *What did you eat today?*

BREAKFAST: ....

Snack: ....

LUNCH: ....

Snack: ....

DINNER: ....

Snack: ....

DRINK: *What did you drink today?*

Any caffeinated drinks: ....

Any alcoholic drinks: ....

Any other drinks: ....

Any other drugs ingested: (including prescription, recreational, over the counter and nicotine) ....

....

QUICK CHECKLIST

WATER - how many litres? ▨   MEDITATION - how many minutes? ▨

SLEEP - how many hours? ▨   EXERCISE - how many minutes? ▨

LIFE EVENTS: *What happened today?*

....

....

....

EMOTIONS/THOUGHTS: *How did you feel today?*

....

....

....

CONCERNS LIST: *What bothered you most today?*

....

....

....

GRATITUDE LIST: *What are you most grateful for today?*

....

....

....

DATE .... **YEAR** ....

FOOD: *What did you eat today?*

BREAKFAST: ....

Snack: ....

LUNCH: ....

Snack: ....

DINNER: ....

Snack: ....

DRINK: *What did you drink today?*

Any caffeinated drinks: ....

Any alcoholic drinks: ....

Any other drinks: ....

Any other drugs ingested: (including prescription, recreational, over the counter and nicotine) ....

....

QUICK CHECKLIST

WATER - how many litres? ⬜   MEDITATION - how many minutes? ⬜

SLEEP - how many hours? ⬜   EXERCISE - how many minutes? ⬜

LIFE EVENTS: *What happened today?*

....

....

....

EMOTIONS/THOUGHTS: *How did you feel today?*

....

....

....

CONCERNS LIST: *What bothered you most today?*

....

....

....

GRATITUDE LIST: *What are you most grateful for today?*

....

....

....

DATE .... **YEAR** ....

FOOD: *What did you eat today?*

BREAKFAST: ....

Snack: ....

LUNCH: ....

Snack: ....

DINNER: ....

Snack: ....

DRINK: *What did you drink today?*

Any caffeinated drinks: ....

Any alcoholic drinks: ....

Any other drinks: ....

Any other drugs ingested: (including prescription, recreational, over the counter and nicotine) ....

....

QUICK CHECKLIST

WATER - how many litres? ▓   MEDITATION - how many minutes? ▓

SLEEP - how many hours? ▓   EXERCISE - how many minutes? ▓

LIFE EVENTS: *What happened today?*

....

....

....

EMOTIONS/THOUGHTS: *How did you feel today?*

....

....

....

CONCERNS LIST: *What bothered you most today?*

....

....

....

GRATITUDE LIST: *What are you most grateful for today?*

....

....

....

DATE .... **YEAR** ....

FOOD: *What did you eat today?*

BREAKFAST: ....

Snack: ....

LUNCH: ....

Snack: ....

DINNER: ....

Snack: ....

DRINK: *What did you drink today?*

Any caffeinated drinks: ....

Any alcoholic drinks: ....

Any other drinks: ....

Any other drugs ingested: (including prescription, recreational, over the counter and nicotine) ....

....

QUICK CHECKLIST

WATER - how many litres? ▢   MEDITATION - how many minutes? ▢

SLEEP - how many hours? ▢   EXERCISE - how many minutes? ▢

LIFE EVENTS: *What happened today?*

....

....

....

EMOTIONS/THOUGHTS: *How did you feel today?*

....

....

....

CONCERNS LIST: *What bothered you most today?*

....

....

....

GRATITUDE LIST: *What are you most grateful for today?*

....

....

....

DATE .... **YEAR** ....

FOOD: *What did you eat today?*

BREAKFAST: ....

Snack: ....

LUNCH: ....

Snack: ....

DINNER: ....

Snack: ....

DRINK: *What did you drink today?*

Any caffeinated drinks: ....

Any alcoholic drinks: ....

Any other drinks: ....

Any other drugs ingested: (including prescription, recreational, over the counter and nicotine) ....

....

QUICK CHECKLIST

WATER - how many litres? ☐   MEDITATION - how many minutes? ☐

SLEEP - how many hours? ☐   EXERCISE - how many minutes? ☐

LIFE EVENTS: *What happened today?*

....

....

....

EMOTIONS/THOUGHTS: *How did you feel today?*

....

....

....

CONCERNS LIST: *What bothered you most today?*

....

....

....

GRATITUDE LIST: *What are you most grateful for today?*

....

....

....

DATE .... **YEAR** ....

FOOD: *What did you eat today?*

BREAKFAST: ....

Snack: ....

LUNCH: ....

Snack: ....

DINNER: ....

Snack: ....

DRINK: *What did you drink today?*

Any caffeinated drinks: ....

Any alcoholic drinks: ....

Any other drinks: ....

Any other drugs ingested: (including prescription, recreational, over the counter and nicotine) ....

....

QUICK CHECKLIST

WATER - how many litres? ☐   MEDITATION - how many minutes? ☐

SLEEP - how many hours? ☐   EXERCISE - how many minutes? ☐

LIFE EVENTS: *What happened today?*

....

....

....

EMOTIONS/THOUGHTS: *How did you feel today?*

....

....

....

CONCERNS LIST: *What bothered you most today?*

....

....

....

GRATITUDE LIST: *What are you most grateful for today?*

....

....

....

DATE .... **YEAR** ....

FOOD: *What did you eat today?*

BREAKFAST: ....

Snack: ....

LUNCH: ....

Snack: ....

DINNER: ....

Snack: ....

DRINK: *What did you drink today?*

Any caffeinated drinks: ....

Any alcoholic drinks: ....

Any other drinks: ....

Any other drugs ingested: (including prescription, recreational, over the counter and nicotine) ....

....

QUICK CHECKLIST

WATER - how many litres?   ▦   MEDITATION - how many minutes?   ▦

SLEEP - how many hours?   ▦   EXERCISE - how many minutes?   ▦

LIFE EVENTS: *What happened today?*

....

....

....

EMOTIONS/THOUGHTS: *How did you feel today?*

....

....

....

CONCERNS LIST: *What bothered you most today?*

....

....

....

GRATITUDE LIST: *What are you most grateful for today?*

....

....

....

DATE .... **YEAR** ....

FOOD: *What did you eat today?*

BREAKFAST: ....

Snack: ....

LUNCH: ....

Snack: ....

DINNER: ....

Snack: ....

DRINK: *What did you drink today?*

Any caffeinated drinks: ....

Any alcoholic drinks: ....

Any other drinks: ....

Any other drugs ingested: (including prescription, recreational, over the counter and nicotine) ....

....

QUICK CHECKLIST

WATER - how many litres? ☐   MEDITATION - how many minutes? ☐

SLEEP - how many hours? ☐   EXERCISE - how many minutes? ☐

LIFE EVENTS: *What happened today?*

....

....

....

EMOTIONS/THOUGHTS: *How did you feel today?*

....

....

....

CONCERNS LIST: *What bothered you most today?*

....

....

....

GRATITUDE LIST: *What are you most grateful for today?*

....

....

....

DATE .... YEAR ....

FOOD: *What did you eat today?*

BREAKFAST: ....

Snack: ....

LUNCH: ....

Snack: ....

DINNER: ....

Snack: ....

DRINK: *What did you drink today?*

Any caffeinated drinks: ....

Any alcoholic drinks: ....

Any other drinks: ....

Any other drugs ingested: (including prescription, recreational, over the counter and nicotine) ....

....

QUICK CHECKLIST

WATER - how many litres? ▢   MEDITATION - how many minutes? ▢

SLEEP - how many hours? ▢   EXERCISE - how many minutes? ▢

LIFE EVENTS: *What happened today?*

....

....

....

EMOTIONS/THOUGHTS: *How did you feel today?*

....

....

....

CONCERNS LIST: *What bothered you most today?*

....

....

....

GRATITUDE LIST: *What are you most grateful for today?*

....

....

....

DATE .... **YEAR** ....

FOOD: *What did you eat today?*

BREAKFAST: ....

Snack: ....

LUNCH: ....

Snack: ....

DINNER: ....

Snack: ....

DRINK: *What did you drink today?*

Any caffeinated drinks: ....

Any alcoholic drinks: ....

Any other drinks: ....

Any other drugs ingested: (including prescription, recreational, over the counter and nicotine) ....

....

QUICK CHECKLIST

WATER - how many litres? ▢   MEDITATION - how many minutes? ▢

SLEEP - how many hours? ▢   EXERCISE - how many minutes? ▢

LIFE EVENTS: *What happened today?*

....

....

....

EMOTIONS/THOUGHTS: *How did you feel today?*

....

....

....

CONCERNS LIST: *What bothered you most today?*

....

....

....

GRATITUDE LIST: *What are you most grateful for today?*

....

....

....

DATE .... **YEAR** ....

FOOD: *What did you eat today?*

BREAKFAST: ....

Snack: ....

LUNCH: ....

Snack: ....

DINNER: ....

Snack: ....

DRINK: *What did you drink today?*

Any caffeinated drinks: ....

Any alcoholic drinks: ....

Any other drinks: ....

Any other drugs ingested: (including prescription, recreational, over the counter and nicotine) ....

....

QUICK CHECKLIST

WATER - how many litres? ▨   MEDITATION - how many minutes? ▨

SLEEP - how many hours? ▨   EXERCISE - how many minutes? ▨

LIFE EVENTS: *What happened today?*

....

....

....

EMOTIONS/THOUGHTS: *How did you feel today?*

....

....

....

CONCERNS LIST: *What bothered you most today?*

....

....

....

GRATITUDE LIST: *What are you most grateful for today?*

....

....

....

DATE .... **YEAR** ....

FOOD: *What did you eat today?*

BREAKFAST: ....

Snack: ....

LUNCH: ....

Snack: ....

DINNER: ....

Snack: ....

DRINK: *What did you drink today?*

Any caffeinated drinks: ....

Any alcoholic drinks: ....

Any other drinks: ....

Any other drugs ingested: (including prescription, recreational, over the counter and nicotine) ....

....

QUICK CHECKLIST

WATER - how many litres? ▩   MEDITATION - how many minutes? ▩

SLEEP - how many hours? ▩   EXERCISE - how many minutes? ▩

LIFE EVENTS: *What happened today?*

....

....

....

EMOTIONS/THOUGHTS: *How did you feel today?*

....

....

....

CONCERNS LIST: *What bothered you most today?*

....

....

....

GRATITUDE LIST: *What are you most grateful for today?*

....

....

....

DATE .... **YEAR** ....

FOOD: *What did you eat today?*

BREAKFAST: ....

Snack: ....

LUNCH: ....

Snack: ....

DINNER: ....

Snack: ....

DRINK: *What did you drink today?*

Any caffeinated drinks: ....

Any alcoholic drinks: ....

Any other drinks: ....

Any other drugs ingested: (including prescription, recreational, over the counter and nicotine) ....

....

QUICK CHECKLIST

WATER - how many litres? ▢   MEDITATION - how many minutes? ▢

SLEEP - how many hours? ▢   EXERCISE - how many minutes? ▢

LIFE EVENTS: *What happened today?*

....

....

....

EMOTIONS/THOUGHTS: *How did you feel today?*

....

....

....

CONCERNS LIST: *What bothered you most today?*

....

....

....

GRATITUDE LIST: *What are you most grateful for today?*

....

....

....

DATE .... **YEAR** ....

FOOD: *What did you eat today?*

BREAKFAST: ....

Snack: ....

LUNCH: ....

Snack: ....

DINNER: ....

Snack: ....

DRINK: *What did you drink today?*

Any caffeinated drinks: ....

Any alcoholic drinks: ....

Any other drinks: ....

Any other drugs ingested: (including prescription, recreational, over the counter and nicotine) ....

....

QUICK CHECKLIST

WATER - how many litres? ⬜   MEDITATION - how many minutes? ⬜

SLEEP - how many hours? ⬜   EXERCISE - how many minutes? ⬜

LIFE EVENTS: *What happened today?*

....

....

....

EMOTIONS/THOUGHTS: *How did you feel today?*

....

....

....

CONCERNS LIST: *What bothered you most today?*

....

....

....

GRATITUDE LIST: *What are you most grateful for today?*

....

....

....

DATE .... **YEAR** ....

FOOD: *What did you eat today?*

BREAKFAST: ....

Snack: ....

LUNCH: ....

Snack: ....

DINNER: ....

Snack: ....

DRINK: *What did you drink today?*

Any caffeinated drinks: ....

Any alcoholic drinks: ....

Any other drinks: ....

Any other drugs ingested: (including prescription, recreational, over the counter and nicotine) ....

....

QUICK CHECKLIST

WATER - how many litres? ▢   MEDITATION - how many minutes? ▢

SLEEP - how many hours? ▢   EXERCISE - how many minutes? ▢

LIFE EVENTS: *What happened today?*

....

....

....

EMOTIONS/THOUGHTS: *How did you feel today?*

....

....

....

CONCERNS LIST: *What bothered you most today?*

....

....

....

GRATITUDE LIST: *What are you most grateful for today?*

....

....

....

DATE .... **YEAR** ....

FOOD: *What did you eat today?*

BREAKFAST: ....

Snack: ....

LUNCH: ....

Snack: ....

DINNER: ....

Snack: ....

DRINK: *What did you drink today?*

Any caffeinated drinks: ....

Any alcoholic drinks: ....

Any other drinks: ....

Any other drugs ingested: (including prescription, recreational, over the counter and nicotine) ....

....

QUICK CHECKLIST

WATER - how many litres? ▨   MEDITATION - how many minutes? ▨

SLEEP - how many hours? ▨   EXERCISE - how many minutes? ▨

LIFE EVENTS: *What happened today?*

....

....

....

EMOTIONS/THOUGHTS: *How did you feel today?*

....

....

....

CONCERNS LIST: *What bothered you most today?*

....

....

....

GRATITUDE LIST: *What are you most grateful for today?*

....

....

....

DATE .... **YEAR** ....

FOOD: *What did you eat today?*

BREAKFAST: ....

Snack: ....

LUNCH: ....

Snack: ....

DINNER: ....

Snack: ....

DRINK: *What did you drink today?*

Any caffeinated drinks: ....

Any alcoholic drinks: ....

Any other drinks: ....

Any other drugs ingested: (including prescription, recreational, over the counter and nicotine) ....

....

QUICK CHECKLIST

WATER - how many litres? ☐   MEDITATION - how many minutes? ☐

SLEEP - how many hours? ☐   EXERCISE - how many minutes? ☐

LIFE EVENTS: *What happened today?*

....

....

....

EMOTIONS/THOUGHTS: *How did you feel today?*

....

....

....

CONCERNS LIST: *What bothered you most today?*

....

....

....

GRATITUDE LIST: *What are you most grateful for today?*

....

....

....

MONTH

TWELVE

mindfulness, meditation and breathing

Being mindful means to feel completely present in the moment you're living in. Aware of your thoughts, emotions and experiences but not feeling anxiously attached to outcomes or expectations. To practice mindfulness, try to maintain a calm curiosity rather than any sort of judgemental attitude. Try to appreciate every sensation as you experience it; appreciating that everything is transient. When we fully value the moment we're in, we can feel profoundly grateful for our lives. We are more able to treasure the good times, withstand the bad and make the most of every opportunity.

Introducing a meditation practice to your daily routine is one of the best ways to make time for yourself. You don't have to spend hours meditation to get results. Studies have shown that spending just five minutes every day, sitting quietly, breathing evenly and calming your mind has a hugely positive impact on physical and mental health. Try doing this before you even get out of bed in the morning. Try choosing a positive affirmation from the back of this book, there's are 365 different suggestions, one for each day of the year, and focus on that thought as you breathe in and out. People who try this practice, for even just one month, routinely report back with amazing positive shifts in their outlooks.

With regards to how you breathe, obviously breathing is fairly important. Every cell in your body is dependent on oxygen and this is achieved by breathing, but it's an automatic process. We don't have to think about it for it to happen. It's meant to occur naturally without conscious interference from us. When we're stressed or anxious however, we *do* interfere with it - we tend to breathe in a way that's fast, shallow and irregular. This causes discomfort and distress both physically and mentally. When our breathing feels laboured, we become aware of it and that increases anxiety and we can get trapped in a cycle.

When we're calm, we breathe slowly, deeply and rhythmically, which in turn promotes a sense of well-being and relaxation. That's why breathing techniques are regularly advocated for unwinding. Anatomically, there is a favourable equilibrium with regards to breathing and we do it naturally when we're at our most relaxed. Unfortunately, this can be easily disrupted by many things: stress, anxiety, depression, sleep deprivation, drug use, illness and even just an unnatural hyper-awareness of our own breath. So just aim for being calm, mindful and relaxed and your breathing will take care of itself.

MONTH .... YEAR ....

Diet

	1	2	3	4	5	6	7	8	9	10	11	12	13	14	15	16	17	18	19	20	21	22	23	24	25	26	27	28	29	30	31
+3																															
+2																															
+1																															
1																															
-2																															
-3																															

Exercise

	1	2	3	4	5	6	7	8	9	10	11	12	13	14	15	16	17	18	19	20	21	22	23	24	25	26	27	28	29	30	31
+3																															
+2																															
+1																															
-1																															
-2																															
-3																															

Life Events

	1	2	3	4	5	6	7	8	9	10	11	12	13	14	15	16	17	18	19	20	21	22	23	24	25	26	27	28	29	30	31
+3																															
+2																															
+1																															
-1																															
-2																															
-3																															

Emotions

	1	2	3	4	5	6	7	8	9	10	11	12	13	14	15	16	17	18	19	20	21	22	23	24	25	26	27	28	29	30	31
+3																															
+2																															
+1																															
-1																															
-2																															
-3																															

Your Choice

	1	2	3	4	5	6	7	8	9	10	11	12	13	14	15	16	17	18	19	20	21	22	23	24	25	26	27	28	29	30	31
+3																															
+2																															
+1																															
-1																															
-2																															
-3																															

Additional Influences   A ....   **B** ....

A	1	2	3	4	5	6	7	8	9	10	11	12	13	14	15	16	17	18	19	20	21	22	23	24	25	26	27	28	29	30	31

B	1	2	3	4	5	6	7	8	9	10	11	12	13	14	15	16	17	18	19	20	21	22	23	24	25	26	27	28	29	30	31

DATE .... **YEAR** ....

FOOD: *What did you eat today?*

BREAKFAST: ....

Snack: ....

LUNCH: ....

Snack: ....

DINNER: ....

Snack: ....

DRINK: *What did you drink today?*

Any caffeinated drinks: ....

Any alcoholic drinks: ....

Any other drinks: ....

Any other drugs ingested: (including prescription, recreational, over the counter and nicotine) ....

....

QUICK CHECKLIST

WATER - how many litres? ▢   MEDITATION - how many minutes? ▢

SLEEP - how many hours? ▢   EXERCISE - how many minutes? ▢

LIFE EVENTS: *What happened today?*

....

....

....

EMOTIONS/THOUGHTS: *How did you feel today?*

....

....

....

CONCERNS LIST: *What bothered you most today?*

....

....

....

GRATITUDE LIST: *What are you most grateful for today?*

....

....

....

DATE .... **YEAR** ....

FOOD: *What did you eat today?*

BREAKFAST: ....

Snack: ....

LUNCH: ....

Snack: ....

DINNER: ....

Snack: ....

DRINK: *What did you drink today?*

Any caffeinated drinks: ....

Any alcoholic drinks: ....

Any other drinks: ....

Any other drugs ingested: (including prescription, recreational, over the counter and nicotine) ....

....

QUICK CHECKLIST

WATER - how many litres? ☐   MEDITATION - how many minutes? ☐

SLEEP - how many hours? ☐   EXERCISE - how many minutes? ☐

LIFE EVENTS: *What happened today?*

....

....

....

EMOTIONS/THOUGHTS: *How did you feel today?*

....

....

....

CONCERNS LIST: *What bothered you most today?*

....

....

....

GRATITUDE LIST: *What are you most grateful for today?*

....

....

....

DATE .... YEAR ....

FOOD: *What did you eat today?*

BREAKFAST: ....

Snack: ....

LUNCH: ....

Snack: ....

DINNER: ....

Snack: ....

DRINK: *What did you drink today?*

Any caffeinated drinks: ....

Any alcoholic drinks: ....

Any other drinks: ....

Any other drugs ingested: (including prescription, recreational, over the counter and nicotine) ....

....

QUICK CHECKLIST

WATER - how many litres? ☐   MEDITATION - how many minutes? ☐

SLEEP - how many hours? ☐   EXERCISE - how many minutes? ☐

LIFE EVENTS: *What happened today?*

....

....

....

EMOTIONS/THOUGHTS: *How did you feel today?*

....

....

....

CONCERNS LIST: *What bothered you most today?*

....

....

....

GRATITUDE LIST: *What are you most grateful for today?*

....

....

....

DATE .... **YEAR** ....

FOOD: *What did you eat today?*

BREAKFAST: ....

Snack: ....

LUNCH: ....

Snack: ....

DINNER: ....

Snack: ....

DRINK: *What did you drink today?*

Any caffeinated drinks: ....

Any alcoholic drinks: ....

Any other drinks: ....

Any other drugs ingested: (including prescription, recreational, over the counter and nicotine) ....

....

QUICK CHECKLIST

WATER - how many litres? ☐   MEDITATION - how many minutes? ☐

SLEEP - how many hours? ☐   EXERCISE - how many minutes? ☐

LIFE EVENTS: *What happened today?*

....

....

....

EMOTIONS/THOUGHTS: *How did you feel today?*

....

....

....

CONCERNS LIST: *What bothered you most today?*

....

....

....

GRATITUDE LIST: *What are you most grateful for today?*

....

....

....

DATE .... **YEAR** ....

FOOD: *What did you eat today?*

BREAKFAST: ....

Snack: ....

LUNCH: ....

Snack: ....

DINNER: ....

Snack: ....

DRINK: *What did you drink today?*

Any caffeinated drinks: ....

Any alcoholic drinks: ....

Any other drinks: ....

Any other drugs ingested: (including prescription, recreational, over the counter and nicotine) ....

....

QUICK CHECKLIST

WATER - how many litres? ▨   MEDITATION - how many minutes? ▨

SLEEP - how many hours? ▨   EXERCISE - how many minutes? ▨

LIFE EVENTS: *What happened today?*

....

....

....

EMOTIONS/THOUGHTS: *How did you feel today?*

....

....

....

CONCERNS LIST: *What bothered you most today?*

....

....

....

GRATITUDE LIST: *What are you most grateful for today?*

....

....

....

DATE .... **YEAR** ....

FOOD: *What did you eat today?*

BREAKFAST: ....

Snack: ....

LUNCH: ....

Snack: ....

DINNER: ....

Snack: ....

DRINK: *What did you drink today?*

Any caffeinated drinks: ....

Any alcoholic drinks: ....

Any other drinks: ....

Any other drugs ingested: (including prescription, recreational, over the counter and nicotine) ....

....

QUICK CHECKLIST

WATER - how many litres? ▢   MEDITATION - how many minutes? ▢

SLEEP - how many hours? ▢   EXERCISE - how many minutes? ▢

LIFE EVENTS: *What happened today?*

....

....

....

EMOTIONS/THOUGHTS: *How did you feel today?*

....

....

....

CONCERNS LIST: *What bothered you most today?*

....

....

....

GRATITUDE LIST: *What are you most grateful for today?*

....

....

....

DATE .... **YEAR** ....

FOOD: *What did you eat today?*

BREAKFAST: ....

Snack: ....

LUNCH: ....

Snack: ....

DINNER: ....

Snack: ....

DRINK: *What did you drink today?*

Any caffeinated drinks: ....

Any alcoholic drinks: ....

Any other drinks: ....

Any other drugs ingested: (including prescription, recreational, over the counter and nicotine) ....

....

QUICK CHECKLIST

WATER - how many litres? ☐ MEDITATION - how many minutes? ☐

SLEEP - how many hours? ☐ EXERCISE - how many minutes? ☐

LIFE EVENTS: *What happened today?*

....

....

....

EMOTIONS/THOUGHTS: *How did you feel today?*

....

....

....

CONCERNS LIST: *What bothered you most today?*

....

....

....

GRATITUDE LIST: *What are you most grateful for today?*

....

....

....

DATE .... **YEAR** ....

FOOD: *What did you eat today?*

BREAKFAST: ....

Snack: ....

LUNCH: ....

Snack: ....

DINNER: ....

Snack: ....

DRINK: *What did you drink today?*

Any caffeinated drinks: ....

Any alcoholic drinks: ....

Any other drinks: ....

Any other drugs ingested: (including prescription, recreational, over the counter and nicotine) ....

....

QUICK CHECKLIST

WATER - how many litres? ▨   MEDITATION - how many minutes? ▨

SLEEP - how many hours? ▨   EXERCISE - how many minutes? ▨

LIFE EVENTS: *What happened today?*

....

....

....

EMOTIONS/THOUGHTS: *How did you feel today?*

....

....

....

CONCERNS LIST: *What bothered you most today?*

....

....

....

GRATITUDE LIST: *What are you most grateful for today?*

....

....

....

DATE .... **YEAR** ....

FOOD: *What did you eat today?*

BREAKFAST: ....

Snack: ....

LUNCH: ....

Snack: ....

DINNER: ....

Snack: ....

DRINK: *What did you drink today?*

Any caffeinated drinks: ....

Any alcoholic drinks: ....

Any other drinks: ....

Any other drugs ingested: (including prescription, recreational, over the counter and nicotine) ....

....

QUICK CHECKLIST

WATER - how many litres? ▨   MEDITATION - how many minutes? ▨

SLEEP - how many hours? ▨   EXERCISE - how many minutes? ▨

LIFE EVENTS: *What happened today?*

....

....

....

EMOTIONS/THOUGHTS: *How did you feel today?*

....

....

....

CONCERNS LIST: *What bothered you most today?*

....

....

....

GRATITUDE LIST: *What are you most grateful for today?*

....

....

....

DATE .... **YEAR** ....

FOOD: *What did you eat today?*

BREAKFAST: ....

Snack: ....

LUNCH: ....

Snack: ....

DINNER: ....

Snack: ....

DRINK: *What did you drink today?*

Any caffeinated drinks: ....

Any alcoholic drinks: ....

Any other drinks: ....

Any other drugs ingested: (including prescription, recreational, over the counter and nicotine) ....

....

QUICK CHECKLIST

WATER - how many litres? ☐   MEDITATION - how many minutes? ☐

SLEEP - how many hours? ☐   EXERCISE - how many minutes? ☐

LIFE EVENTS: *What happened today?*

....

....

....

EMOTIONS/THOUGHTS: *How did you feel today?*

....

....

....

CONCERNS LIST: *What bothered you most today?*

....

....

....

GRATITUDE LIST: *What are you most grateful for today?*

....

....

....

DATE .... **YEAR** ....

FOOD: *What did you eat today?*

BREAKFAST: ....

Snack: ....

LUNCH: ....

Snack: ....

DINNER: ....

Snack: ....

DRINK: *What did you drink today?*

Any caffeinated drinks: ....

Any alcoholic drinks: ....

Any other drinks: ....

Any other drugs ingested: (including prescription, recreational, over the counter and nicotine) ....

....

QUICK CHECKLIST

WATER - how many litres? ▢   MEDITATION - how many minutes? ▢

SLEEP - how many hours? ▢   EXERCISE - how many minutes? ▢

LIFE EVENTS: *What happened today?*

....

....

....

EMOTIONS/THOUGHTS: *How did you feel today?*

....

....

....

CONCERNS LIST: *What bothered you most today?*

....

....

....

GRATITUDE LIST: *What are you most grateful for today?*

....

....

....

DATE .... **YEAR** ....

FOOD: *What did you eat today?*

BREAKFAST: ....

Snack: ....

LUNCH: ....

Snack: ....

DINNER: ....

Snack: ....

DRINK: *What did you drink today?*

Any caffeinated drinks: ....

Any alcoholic drinks: ....

Any other drinks: ....

Any other drugs ingested: (including prescription, recreational, over the counter and nicotine) ....

....

QUICK CHECKLIST

WATER - how many litres? ▨   MEDITATION - how many minutes? ▨

SLEEP - how many hours? ▨   EXERCISE - how many minutes? ▨

LIFE EVENTS: *What happened today?*

....

....

....

EMOTIONS/THOUGHTS: *How did you feel today?*

....

....

....

CONCERNS LIST: *What bothered you most today?*

....

....

....

GRATITUDE LIST: *What are you most grateful for today?*

....

....

....

DATE .... **YEAR** ....

FOOD: *What did you eat today?*

BREAKFAST: ....

Snack: ....

LUNCH: ....

Snack: ....

DINNER: ....

Snack: ....

DRINK: *What did you drink today?*

Any caffeinated drinks: ....

Any alcoholic drinks: ....

Any other drinks: ....

Any other drugs ingested: (including prescription, recreational, over the counter and nicotine) ....

....

QUICK CHECKLIST

WATER - how many litres? ▨   MEDITATION - how many minutes? ▨

SLEEP - how many hours? ▨   EXERCISE - how many minutes? ▨

LIFE EVENTS: *What happened today?*

....

....

....

EMOTIONS/THOUGHTS: *How did you feel today?*

....

....

....

CONCERNS LIST: *What bothered you most today?*

....

....

....

GRATITUDE LIST: *What are you most grateful for today?*

....

....

....

DATE .... **YEAR** ....

FOOD: *What did you eat today?*

BREAKFAST: ....

Snack: ....

LUNCH: ....

Snack: ....

DINNER: ....

Snack: ....

DRINK: *What did you drink today?*

Any caffeinated drinks: ....

Any alcoholic drinks: ....

Any other drinks: ....

Any other drugs ingested: (including prescription, recreational, over the counter and nicotine) ....

....

QUICK CHECKLIST

WATER - how many litres? ▨   MEDITATION - how many minutes? ▨

SLEEP - how many hours? ▨   EXERCISE - how many minutes? ▨

LIFE EVENTS: *What happened today?*

....

....

....

EMOTIONS/THOUGHTS: *How did you feel today?*

....

....

....

CONCERNS LIST: *What bothered you most today?*

....

....

....

GRATITUDE LIST: *What are you most grateful for today?*

....

....

....

DATE .... YEAR ....

FOOD: *What did you eat today?*

BREAKFAST: ....

Snack: ....

LUNCH: ....

Snack: ....

DINNER: ....

Snack: ....

DRINK: *What did you drink today?*

Any caffeinated drinks: ....

Any alcoholic drinks: ....

Any other drinks: ....

Any other drugs ingested: (including prescription, recreational, over the counter and nicotine) ....

....

QUICK CHECKLIST

WATER - how many litres? ☐   MEDITATION - how many minutes? ☐

SLEEP - how many hours? ☐   EXERCISE - how many minutes? ☐

LIFE EVENTS: *What happened today?*

....

....

....

EMOTIONS/THOUGHTS: *How did you feel today?*

....

....

....

CONCERNS LIST: *What bothered you most today?*

....

....

....

GRATITUDE LIST: *What are you most grateful for today?*

....

....

....

DATE .... **YEAR** ....

FOOD: *What did you eat today?*

BREAKFAST: ....

Snack: ....

LUNCH: ....

Snack: ....

DINNER: ....

Snack: ....

DRINK: *What did you drink today?*

Any caffeinated drinks: ....

Any alcoholic drinks: ....

Any other drinks: ....

Any other drugs ingested: (including prescription, recreational, over the counter and nicotine) ....

....

QUICK CHECKLIST

WATER - how many litres? ▫   MEDITATION - how many minutes? ▫

SLEEP - how many hours? ▫   EXERCISE - how many minutes? ▫

LIFE EVENTS: *What happened today?*

....

....

....

EMOTIONS/THOUGHTS: *How did you feel today?*

....

....

....

CONCERNS LIST: *What bothered you most today?*

....

....

....

GRATITUDE LIST: *What are you most grateful for today?*

....

....

....

DATE .... YEAR ....

FOOD: *What did you eat today?*

BREAKFAST: ....

Snack: ....

LUNCH: ....

Snack: ....

DINNER: ....

Snack: ....

DRINK: *What did you drink today?*

Any caffeinated drinks: ....

Any alcoholic drinks: ....

Any other drinks: ....

Any other drugs ingested: (including prescription, recreational, over the counter and nicotine) ....

....

QUICK CHECKLIST

WATER - how many litres? ▨   MEDITATION - how many minutes? ▨

SLEEP - how many hours? ▨   EXERCISE - how many minutes? ▨

LIFE EVENTS: *What happened today?*

....

....

....

EMOTIONS/THOUGHTS: *How did you feel today?*

....

....

....

CONCERNS LIST: *What bothered you most today?*

....

....

....

GRATITUDE LIST: *What are you most grateful for today?*

....

....

....

DATE .... **YEAR** ....

FOOD: *What did you eat today?*

BREAKFAST: ....

Snack: ....

LUNCH: ....

Snack: ....

DINNER: ....

Snack: ....

DRINK: *What did you drink today?*

Any caffeinated drinks: ....

Any alcoholic drinks: ....

Any other drinks: ....

Any other drugs ingested: (including prescription, recreational, over the counter and nicotine) ....

....

QUICK CHECKLIST

WATER - how many litres? ▢   MEDITATION - how many minutes? ▢

SLEEP - how many hours? ▢   EXERCISE - how many minutes? ▢

LIFE EVENTS: *What happened today?*

....

....

....

EMOTIONS/THOUGHTS: *How did you feel today?*

....

....

....

CONCERNS LIST: *What bothered you most today?*

....

....

....

GRATITUDE LIST: *What are you most grateful for today?*

....

....

....

DATE .... **YEAR** ....

FOOD: *What did you eat today?*

BREAKFAST: ....

Snack: ....

LUNCH: ....

Snack: ....

DINNER: ....

Snack: ....

DRINK: *What did you drink today?*

Any caffeinated drinks: ....

Any alcoholic drinks: ....

Any other drinks: ....

Any other drugs ingested: (including prescription, recreational, over the counter and nicotine) ....

....

QUICK CHECKLIST

WATER - how many litres? ☐   MEDITATION - how many minutes? ☐

SLEEP - how many hours? ☐   EXERCISE - how many minutes? ☐

LIFE EVENTS: *What happened today?*

....

....

....

EMOTIONS/THOUGHTS: *How did you feel today?*

....

....

....

CONCERNS LIST: *What bothered you most today?*

....

....

....

GRATITUDE LIST: *What are you most grateful for today?*

....

....

....

DATE .... **YEAR** ....

FOOD: *What did you eat today?*

BREAKFAST: ....

Snack: ....

LUNCH: ....

Snack: ....

DINNER: ....

Snack: ....

DRINK: *What did you drink today?*

Any caffeinated drinks: ....

Any alcoholic drinks: ....

Any other drinks: ....

Any other drugs ingested: (including prescription, recreational, over the counter and nicotine) ....

....

QUICK CHECKLIST

WATER - how many litres? ▢   MEDITATION - how many minutes? ▢

SLEEP - how many hours? ▢   EXERCISE - how many minutes? ▢

LIFE EVENTS: *What happened today?*

....

....

....

EMOTIONS/THOUGHTS: *How did you feel today?*

....

....

....

CONCERNS LIST: *What bothered you most today?*

....

....

....

GRATITUDE LIST: *What are you most grateful for today?*

....

....

....

DATE .... **YEAR** ....

FOOD: *What did you eat today?*

BREAKFAST: ....

Snack: ....

LUNCH: ....

Snack: ....

DINNER: ....

Snack: ....

DRINK: *What did you drink today?*

Any caffeinated drinks: ....

Any alcoholic drinks: ....

Any other drinks: ....

Any other drugs ingested: (including prescription, recreational, over the counter and nicotine) ....

....

QUICK CHECKLIST

WATER - how many litres? ☐   MEDITATION - how many minutes? ☐

SLEEP - how many hours? ☐   EXERCISE - how many minutes? ☐

LIFE EVENTS: *What happened today?*

....

....

....

EMOTIONS/THOUGHTS: *How did you feel today?*

....

....

....

CONCERNS LIST: *What bothered you most today?*

....

....

....

GRATITUDE LIST: *What are you most grateful for today?*

....

....

....

DATE .... **YEAR** ....

FOOD: *What did you eat today?*

BREAKFAST: ....

Snack: ....

LUNCH: ....

Snack: ....

DINNER: ....

Snack: ....

DRINK: *What did you drink today?*

Any caffeinated drinks: ....

Any alcoholic drinks: ....

Any other drinks: ....

Any other drugs ingested: (including prescription, recreational, over the counter and nicotine) ....

....

QUICK CHECKLIST

WATER - how many litres? ☐   MEDITATION - how many minutes? ☐

SLEEP - how many hours? ☐   EXERCISE - how many minutes? ☐

LIFE EVENTS: *What happened today?*

....

....

....

EMOTIONS/THOUGHTS: *How did you feel today?*

....

....

....

CONCERNS LIST: *What bothered you most today?*

....

....

....

GRATITUDE LIST: *What are you most grateful for today?*

....

....

....

DATE .... **YEAR** ....

FOOD: *What did you eat today?*

BREAKFAST: ....

Snack: ....

LUNCH: ....

Snack: ....

DINNER: ....

Snack: ....

DRINK: *What did you drink today?*

Any caffeinated drinks: ....

Any alcoholic drinks: ....

Any other drinks: ....

Any other drugs ingested: (including prescription, recreational, over the counter and nicotine) ....

....

QUICK CHECKLIST

WATER - how many litres? ▢   MEDITATION - how many minutes? ▢

SLEEP - how many hours? ▢   EXERCISE - how many minutes? ▢

LIFE EVENTS: *What happened today?*

....

....

....

EMOTIONS/THOUGHTS: *How did you feel today?*

....

....

....

CONCERNS LIST: *What bothered you most today?*

....

....

....

GRATITUDE LIST: *What are you most grateful for today?*

....

....

....

DATE .... **YEAR** ....

FOOD: *What did you eat today?*

BREAKFAST: ....

Snack: ....

LUNCH: ....

Snack: ....

DINNER: ....

Snack: ....

DRINK: *What did you drink today?*

Any caffeinated drinks: ....

Any alcoholic drinks: ....

Any other drinks: ....

Any other drugs ingested: (including prescription, recreational, over the counter and nicotine) ....

....

QUICK CHECKLIST

WATER - how many litres?　▢　　MEDITATION - how many minutes?　▢

SLEEP - how many hours?　▢　　EXERCISE - how many minutes?　▢

LIFE EVENTS: *What happened today?*

....

....

....

EMOTIONS/THOUGHTS: *How did you feel today?*

....

....

....

CONCERNS LIST: *What bothered you most today?*

....

....

....

GRATITUDE LIST: *What are you most grateful for today?*

....

....

....

DATE .... YEAR ....

FOOD: *What did you eat today?*

BREAKFAST: ....

Snack: ....

LUNCH: ....

Snack: ....

DINNER: ....

Snack: ....

DRINK: *What did you drink today?*

Any caffeinated drinks: ....

Any alcoholic drinks: ....

Any other drinks: ....

Any other drugs ingested: (including prescription, recreational, over the counter and nicotine) ....

....

QUICK CHECKLIST

WATER - how many litres? ▢   MEDITATION - how many minutes? ▢

SLEEP - how many hours? ▢   EXERCISE - how many minutes? ▢

LIFE EVENTS: *What happened today?*

....

....

....

EMOTIONS/THOUGHTS: *How did you feel today?*

....

....

....

CONCERNS LIST: *What bothered you most today?*

....

....

....

GRATITUDE LIST: *What are you most grateful for today?*

....

....

....

DATE .... **YEAR** ....

FOOD: *What did you eat today?*

BREAKFAST: ....

Snack: ....

LUNCH: ....

Snack: ....

DINNER: ....

Snack: ....

DRINK: *What did you drink today?*

Any caffeinated drinks: ....

Any alcoholic drinks: ....

Any other drinks: ....

Any other drugs ingested: (including prescription, recreational, over the counter and nicotine) ....

....

QUICK CHECKLIST

WATER - how many litres? ▓   MEDITATION - how many minutes? ▓

SLEEP - how many hours? ▓   EXERCISE - how many minutes? ▓

LIFE EVENTS: *What happened today?*

....

....

....

EMOTIONS/THOUGHTS: *How did you feel today?*

....

....

....

CONCERNS LIST: *What bothered you most today?*

....

....

....

GRATITUDE LIST: *What are you most grateful for today?*

....

....

....

DATE .... YEAR ....

FOOD: *What did you eat today?*

BREAKFAST: ....

Snack: ....

LUNCH: ....

Snack: ....

DINNER: ....

Snack: ....

DRINK: *What did you drink today?*

Any caffeinated drinks: ....

Any alcoholic drinks: ....

Any other drinks: ....

Any other drugs ingested: (including prescription, recreational, over the counter and nicotine) ....

....

QUICK CHECKLIST

WATER - how many litres? ▢   MEDITATION - how many minutes? ▢

SLEEP - how many hours? ▢   EXERCISE - how many minutes? ▢

LIFE EVENTS: *What happened today?*

....

....

....

EMOTIONS/THOUGHTS: *How did you feel today?*

....

....

....

CONCERNS LIST: *What bothered you most today?*

....

....

....

GRATITUDE LIST: *What are you most grateful for today?*

....

....

....

DATE .... **YEAR** ....

FOOD: *What did you eat today?*

BREAKFAST: ....

Snack: ....

LUNCH: ....

Snack: ....

DINNER: ....

Snack: ....

DRINK: *What did you drink today?*

Any caffeinated drinks: ....

Any alcoholic drinks: ....

Any other drinks: ....

Any other drugs ingested: (including prescription, recreational, over the counter and nicotine) ....

....

QUICK CHECKLIST

WATER - how many litres? ▢   MEDITATION - how many minutes? ▢

SLEEP - how many hours? ▢   EXERCISE - how many minutes? ▢

LIFE EVENTS: *What happened today?*

....

....

....

EMOTIONS/THOUGHTS: *How did you feel today?*

....

....

....

CONCERNS LIST: *What bothered you most today?*

....

....

....

GRATITUDE LIST: *What are you most grateful for today?*

....

....

....

DATE .... **YEAR** ....

FOOD: *What did you eat today?*

BREAKFAST: ....

Snack: ....

LUNCH: ....

Snack: ....

DINNER: ....

Snack: ....

DRINK: *What did you drink today?*

Any caffeinated drinks: ....

Any alcoholic drinks: ....

Any other drinks: ....

Any other drugs ingested: (including prescription, recreational, over the counter and nicotine) ....

....

QUICK CHECKLIST

WATER - how many litres? ▢   MEDITATION - how many minutes? ▢

SLEEP - how many hours? ▢   EXERCISE - how many minutes? ▢

LIFE EVENTS: *What happened today?*

....

....

....

EMOTIONS/THOUGHTS: *How did you feel today?*

....

....

....

CONCERNS LIST: *What bothered you most today?*

....

....

....

GRATITUDE LIST: *What are you most grateful for today?*

....

....

....

DATE .... **YEAR** ....

FOOD: *What did you eat today?*

BREAKFAST: ....

Snack: ....

LUNCH: ....

Snack: ....

DINNER: ....

Snack: ....

DRINK: *What did you drink today?*

Any caffeinated drinks: ....

Any alcoholic drinks: ....

Any other drinks: ....

Any other drugs ingested: (including prescription, recreational, over the counter and nicotine) ....

....

QUICK CHECKLIST

WATER - how many litres? ▨   MEDITATION - how many minutes? ▨

SLEEP - how many hours? ▨   EXERCISE - how many minutes? ▨

LIFE EVENTS: *What happened today?*

....

....

....

EMOTIONS/THOUGHTS: *How did you feel today?*

....

....

....

CONCERNS LIST: *What bothered you most today?*

....

....

....

GRATITUDE LIST: *What are you most grateful for today?*

....

....

....

DATE .... **YEAR** ....

FOOD: *What did you eat today?*

BREAKFAST: ....

Snack: ....

LUNCH: ....

Snack: ....

DINNER: ....

Snack: ....

DRINK: *What did you drink today?*

Any caffeinated drinks: ....

Any alcoholic drinks: ....

Any other drinks: ....

Any other drugs ingested: (including prescription, recreational, over the counter and nicotine) ....

....

QUICK CHECKLIST

WATER - how many litres? ☐   MEDITATION - how many minutes? ☐

SLEEP - how many hours? ☐   EXERCISE - how many minutes? ☐

LIFE EVENTS: *What happened today?*

....

....

....

EMOTIONS/THOUGHTS: *How did you feel today?*

....

....

....

CONCERNS LIST: *What bothered you most today?*

....

....

....

GRATITUDE LIST: *What are you most grateful for today?*

....

....

....

<u>positive affirmations</u>

The connection between the mind and body is well established. It's thought that the practice of gently repeating a positive affirmation to yourself each day, even for as little as three minutes, will bring about a powerful shift in your mood. Whenever you start The Off The Rocks Journal, consider also starting a meditation practice from that day forward too. Start at the beginning of this list and work your way through, one day at a time, for a whole year and see how it makes a positive impact on your mental health. Find a quiet place to sit or lie where you won't be interrupted for a few minutes. Read your affirmation for that day and then lovingly and calmly repeat it to yourself, either out loud or in your mind, and just focus on that. Breathe deeply and relax. When other thoughts come into your mind, just observe them and let them go, bringing your attention back to your positive affirmation. Try to do this practice at least once every day for a minimum of five minutes. The more you do this, the more benefit you'll get from it. Get cracking today and good luck!

1. I am full of energy and vitality and my mind is calm and peaceful.
2. I have an attitude of gratitude. I have so much to be grateful for.
3. I am lovely, I am loved, I am loveable.
4. I lovingly nourish my body with healthy food and clean water.
5. I am kind and compassionate to everyone I come into contact with.
6. Every day, in every way, I'm getting better and better.
7. I breathe deeply, exercise regularly and take care of my precious body.
8. I deserve to live a healthy, lovely life.
9. My body is healing itself with every passing second.
10. There is always the opportunity to try again.
11. I can change my life for the better at any moment.
12. I have the power to heal myself.
13. I love feeling happy, healthy and whole.
14. Health, happiness and love are the most important things in life.
15. My body is strong, healthy and beautiful.
16. I forgive what has hurt me and I detach with love.
17. My ability to overcome challenges is limitless.
18. Happiness is a choice and I choose to be happy
19. I effortlessly abandon bad habits and replace them with healthy ones.
20. I am blessed with amazing family and friends.
21. I radiate charm, poise and confidence.

22. I am at total peace with what has happened and what is yet to come.
23. It's a gift to be alive.
24. I already have within me everything that I need.
25. Every decision I make, no matter how small, is made with health in mind.
26. I am never alone, help is all around me if I reach out.
27. I am kind to everyone because I know we all want to feel loved.
28. I feel perfectly content in this exact moment.
29. I am happy and feel enthusiastic about my life.
30. I find pleasure in even the simple things in life.
31. I love to laugh with others.
32. My heart is bursting with happiness.
33. I can't wait to go out today and make someone smile.
34. I easily set healthy boundaries and ensure they're observed.
35. I know that the only person I can change is myself.
36. I love finding new ways to spend my time.
37. I make time every day to practice radical self-care.
38. I know my worth and I respect myself.
39. I communicate calmly, honestly and openly.
40. I wish the very best for people.
41. I give compliments freely and sincerely.
42. I enjoy meeting new people.
43. I am completely comfortable with who I am.
44. I don't take anything personally.
45. It's none of my business what people think of me.
46. I adjust to new situations without any problem.
47. I only see the good in others.
48. I send healing oxygen to every cell in my body with every deep breath.
49. I pay attention to the messages my body sends me.
50. I feel safe, secure, happy and confident.
51. I am excited about the future.
52. I easily let go of the past.
53. I forgive myself as easily as I forgive others.
54. I help others as often as I possibly can.
55. I help myself by helping others.
56. I ask for help whenever I need it and I offer help whenever I can.

57. I respond calmly in every situation.

58. I am responsibly for my own happiness.

59. I happily hold myself accountable for my actions.

60. I focus completely on the task in hand.

61. I am grateful for so much.

62. I find enjoyment at every opportunity.

63. I gently remind myself to keep returning to the present moment.

64. I am strong, loving and powerful beyond measure.

65. My happiness and gratitude knows no bounds.

66. I observe my emotions without becoming attached to them.

67. I release my anxiety with ease.

68. My happiness is unlimited.

69. Being at peace is more important than being right.

70. I treat myself with kindness.

71. I trust my instincts.

72. I know that everything I need is already mine.

73. I've made peace with myself.

74. The better I treat myself, the happier I become.

75. I don't take anything for granted.

76. I am open-minded and don't mind being wrong.

77. I notice the spaces between my thoughts.

78. I know that the behaviour of others is always either an act of love or a call for love.

79. Kindness is my default setting.

80. I am as gentle with myself as I am with others.

81. I can choose my thoughts and I choose them carefully and lovingly.

82. I take small, sure-footed steps every day to take me closer to my goals.

83. I am not afraid, I was born to do this.

84. I easily maintain loving relationships.

85. It is perfectly safe for me to express myself.

86. I am so grateful for everything that I have.

87. I realise how lucky I am.

88. I have everything I could ever wish for.

89. I remember the days when I prayed for what I have now.

90. I don't attach expectations to things. I let outcomes occur naturally.

91. My power lies in being peaceful in the present moment.

92. I see the beauty in everything.

93. I love keeping things simple.

94. I know that a new beginning can start at any time.

95. I appreciate that all experiences are important.

96. I see possibility in all of life's challenges.

97. I look forward to a brand new day.

98. Love and gratitude are the answers to every problem.

99. When I notice that I'm fearful I surrender it fully.

100. I deeply value the opinions of others but know that I don't have to agree.

101. I know it's okay to slow down, relax and let go.

102. I respect the story of my life.

103. I accept whatever happens with dignity and love.

104. At any given moment I can choose a different choice.

105. I pay loving attention to the quality of my thoughts.

106. There is abundance all around me.

107. The energy that I put out comes back to me.

108. Every cell in my body receives my positivity.

109. I believe in infinite possibilities.

110. I am able to take full care of myself.

111. I love my friends and show them that I care.

112. I believe in myself.

113. I trust the evolution of my life.

114. My mind has unlimited power.

115. I make a positive contribution to the world.

116. I lead by my own good example.

117. I love creating new healthy habits.

118. I am grateful to be free of old bad habits.

119. I embrace new challenges because they help me to grow.

120. I see the opportunity in every experience.

121. I work on strengthening a positive mental attitude every single day.

122. I am always in the right place at the right time.

123. Everything is unfolding exactly as it should.

124. I completely trust the process.

125. I have abundant faith in myself.

126. I appreciate the incomprehensible beauty of the universe.

127. I have overcome adversity and it has made me stronger.

128. I strengthen my discipline with each passing second.

129. Every heartbeat is a chance to start again.

130. I am willing to work harder than I have before.

131. I spend my time and energy wisely and lovingly.

132. I can make a different choice any time I want.

133. I am unique and so is everybody else, we are all special in our own ways.

134. I don't have to prove myself to anyone.

135. My happiness doesn't depend on anyone but me.

136. I understand that the more I give, the more I get in return.

137. I know that I need to work on short term goals for long term gains.

138. I have the power and the choice to change my thoughts at any time.

139. I am allowed to do what I want with my own life.

140. The way my body functions and heals itself amazes me.

141. I can do anything I set my mind to.

142. I know, without a doubt, that things do change and can get better.

143. I know that good things can take time and I am happy to be patient.

144. I always learn lessons from my past experiences.

145. Each day has infinite potential and possibility.

146. I show compassion for myself and for all living things.

147. My life is filled with meaning, purpose and passion.

148. I constantly gently bring myself back to the present moment.

149. I accept myself exactly as I am at this moment, I know I'll keep evolving.

150. I understand that now I know better, I can do better.

151. I know that I don't need anyone's approval to make me feel validated.

152. I accept others exactly as they are. It's not my job to change other people.

153. Every problem that arises has a solution.

154. My inner resources are inexhaustible.

155. I always make loving considered decisions. I will not rush myself.

156. All is well, right here, right now.

157. I take my time. There is all the time in the world.

158. I love to organise myself in advance when I can, so I never have to hurry.

159. What others think of me is none of my business.

160. I know what I do today will impact on tomorrow. So I choose wisely.

161. I release myself from any feelings of obligation.

162. I know that worrying doesn't have any positive effects, so I don't worry.

163. I am certain that I can continue being the master of my own emotions.

164. I am stronger than any of my excuses.

165. I trust that things will work out perfectly without any interference.

166. I am capable of doing difficult things.

167. I easily let go of my old self-limiting beliefs.

168. I deserve to feel calm and content and that is in my control.

169. I don't argue with anybody over anything. I know that arguing is futile.

170. I don't allow my fears to stop me from doing anything I want to do.

171. I know that I am a good person. I don't need to defend myself about that.

172. I can accept another point of view without having to agree with it.

173. I know that I don't have to retaliate to anyone about anything.

174. I believe that we are all in this together, trying to do the best we can.

175. Whenever people are mean, I don't take it personally, I wish them well.

176. I set my goals and slowly but surely work towards them.

177. I take one step at a time and that is absolutely enough.

178. I attract the best things for me at exactly the right times.

179. I know that when I change my perception of things, I change my whole life.

180. My inner peace and tranquility cannot be disturbed by anyone but me.

181. I easily resist forming strong attachments to material things.

182. I know that external stimuli is not what governs me.

183. I am immune to the judgement of others. I am robust in my own beliefs.

184. I spend some time every day alone with who I am.

185. I am committed to doing everything I possibly can to promote my health.

186. I identify my personal triggers and I tread gently and respectfully around them.

187. I take responsibility for my actions and apologise whenever necessary.

188. I alleviate my tension in responsible, loving, healthy ways.

189. Until I'm sure of what to do for the best, I try to do nothing.

190. I release anxiety and have faith that I will cope perfectly well.

191. Each and every day, my circumstances are improving.

192. I will remain stable through any challenge.

193. I trust my intuition. I know what is best for me.

194. I choose to behave with absolute honesty and integrity.

195. I extend kindness to everyone I meet.

196. I make choices that reflect how much I care for myself.

197. I try to live sustainably as far as possible. I care deeply about our planet.

198. I accept outcomes with dignity and serenity.

199. I am motivated by love, always.

200. I am willing to forgive because I know that forgiveness sets me free.

201. The past is forgiven and I am thankful for the lessons I've learned.

202. I release all fear from my life.

203. Fear is just a thought. It does not rule my life or control my actions.

204. All of my thoughts are filled with love, peace and tranquility.

205. I am capable of forging amazing friendships.

206. I choose to see the beauty in all things.

207. I have faith that good will overcome.

208. Kindness is everything.

209. I am excited for what today will bring.

210. I treat others how I wish to be treated.

211. I forgive the past so I can be free in the present.

212. I try to find enjoyment in every situation.

213. I consciously choose to focus on all the positive aspects of a situation.

214. Today is another chance to do better than yesterday.

215. Engaging in negativity only perpetuates it. So I don't engage in it.

216. I am happy and excited about being alive.

217. I never engage in gossip. I disengage with compassion and do something better.

218. I express myself fully and freely, I am authentically me.

219. All my needs are being met.

220. There is a way through every situation.

221. My happiness is a choice that I consciously choose over and over again.

222. I release the feeling of struggle. I accept what is.

223. We change our world by changing our perception of the world.

224. I can foster new habits to replace old ones.

225. I make calm considered decisions.

226. I accept what I cannot change.

227. We can't predict the future, so there's no point in worrying about it.

228. The truth means everything. I am truthful in everything I do.

229. I let go of resentments, fears and regrets. I look to a bright future.

230. All the love I have is in my mind.

231. I accept exactly where I am, at exactly this moment.

232. I am energised, I am inspired, I am enthusiastic.

233. I believe I deserve to be happy.

234. I am healing, I am healthy, I am grateful.

235. I don't speak badly about others. Everyone is fighting a battle I know nothing about.

236. I try to leave people happier than when I meet them.

237. I am reliable, I am supportive, I am unwaveringly loyal.

238. I smile often.

239. I know that other people's battles are not mine to fight for them.

240. I easily and lovingly let go of things that no longer serve my highest good.

241. I have fun wherever I go, whatever I do, whoever I'm with.

242. I don't need to compare myself to anybody else. We're all unique.

243. I don't try to control anything or anyone except myself.

244. I change when I change my patterns of behaviour.

245. I am fearless. I've been through worse and survived.

246. I wish good things for everybody.

247. I release myself from any shame.

248. I embrace my experiences, they have made me who I am.

249. Whenever I feel pain, it is trying to tell me something, so I listen.

250. I believe I am capable of profound change.

251. I make self-care a priority. If I don't take care of myself, I can't take care of anyone else.

252. I don't need to change the world; only the way I see it.

253. I am always compassionate towards myself and others.

254. I don't sit in judgement of anybody.

255. Challenging relationships encourage me to look at my own behaviour.

256. My faith is far stronger than my fear.

257. I let go of whatever other people think of me.

258. I am kind and loving to everyone I meet.

259. I know that if I don't like my circumstances, I can change them.

260. I eat food that nourishes and fuels my body.

261. I consistently choose peace over chaos.

262. I have an infinite potential within me that I can access at any time.

263. I know that everything I need to get done will get done at the right time.

264. I work hard to create more of what I want.

265. I don't engage in negativity.

266. I am able to alter my habits the second I become willing.

267. I am endlessly supported and loved.

268. I am complete.

269. I face adversity with courage and grace.

270. I am receptive to new experiences.

271. I care for every single cell in my body.

272. I surround myself with people that I love and admire.

273. The possibilities are endless.

274. I take my good mood with me wherever I go.

275. I love to dance and move my body.

276. I am gentle with myself and feel in touch with my emotions.

277. Optimum health and happiness are my goals.

278. I choose to rise above negativity.

279. I am willing to listen intently to others.

280. I regularly check that my motives are good.

281. I encourage my friends and I am happy for their successes.

282. Tomorrow is another day and another chance to do better.

283. I am wholly committed to living authentically.

284. I am known for telling the truth in a calm, gentle way.

285. It is safe to ask for what I need.

286. It is not my place to sit in judgement of others.

287. I do not doubt myself.

288. I honour myself.

289. I am at perfect ease with myself.

290. I am deeply thankful for everything I have.

291. I am open to change.

292. I care for myself first so I have enough energy left over to care for others.

293. I quickly rebound from adversity.

294. I know that money can't buy love, time, health or happiness.

295. I am genuine in all of my efforts.

296. I am completely trustworthy.

297. I don't berate myself. I treat myself with love and kindness.

298. I am committed to doing the right thing, always.

299. I have the autonomy to do what I like.

300. My contributions matter and are greatly appreciated.

301. I am not afraid to excel.

302. I am capable of creating a beautiful life.

303. Today I will create a beautiful experience.

304. I am protected and guided.

305. I am as happy as I choose to be.

306. I choose my reaction to any given situation.

307. I don't allow my past experiences to define me.

308. I don't attach expectations to anything or anyone.

309. I am good enough.

310. It begins with me.

311. I don't allow criticism to control me.

312. I don't buy what I can't afford.

313. I gently give my body exactly what it needs.

314. I am allowed to change my mind.

315. I respect my own boundaries.

316. I don't assume the worst.

317. I don't hold onto grudges.

318. I make informed decisions.

319. I am unlimited and unstoppable.

320. Other people's perceptions of me don't define me.

321. I learn from my mistakes and I move on from them, graciously taking the lessons with me.

322. I don't assume to know what anyone is thinking.

323. On some level I already have all the answers I need.

324. I treat myself with kindness and consideration.

325. I can heal myself.

326. There is plenty of time to accomplish my goals.

327. I graciously accept help.

328. I attract like-minded friends into my life.

329. I take the time every day to breathe deeply.

330. I can handle any challenge that comes my way.

331. Whenever I sense conflict, I look for my part in it.

332. I diligently work towards my dreams.

333. I walk away from negativity.

334. I trust myself implicitly.

335. I don't let others influence what I do or how I feel.

336. I know that positivity is contagious and I want to help spread it.

337. I gravitate towards inspiring people.

338. I rise above petty concerns.

339. I pay attention to moments of clarity.

340. I am the master of my destiny.

341. How I see things is an indication of how I feel inside.

342. I fully support myself.

343. I feel my feelings fully. I do not try to escape from them.

344. I reach out for help and support when I need to.

345. I am always open to suggestions.

346. Whatever I put out, comes back.

347. I hold myself accountable for the choices I make.

348. I aim for mutual respect in all of my interpersonal relationships.

349. I have nothing to hide.

350. I pay attention to what truly makes me happy.

351. I am brave beyond measure.

352. I give without thought of reward.

353. I am impeccable with my word.

354. I remember not to take things personally.

355. I don't assume to know everything.

356. I always try my best at any given time.

357. I work happily alongside others.

358. I am in alignment with my highest good.

359. I steer clear of danger zones.

360. I know that words are powerful so I choose them carefully.

361. I remember to act with love in every situation I find myself in.

362. I can reframe any situation any time I want.

363. I'm well aware that it's not all about me.

364. I know that we are all connected to each other.

365. I understand that there is infinite love and power within every single one of us.

acknowledgements

Massive thanks to Mommy Nudger, Poppa Doc and Dad; I quite literally wouldn't be here without you. You are the absolute best. My husband, Luke, you are very hot and I love you, in a way.

Big love to all the incredible people who've helped to keep me on track whilst I wrote this book. Your consistent love, loyalty and kindness has never gone unnoticed. Thank you, from the bottom of my heart: Pauline, Kay, Lucy, Ruth, Alexandra, Gabrielle, Steph, Cath, Shelley, Deborah, Lynsey, Mark & Dot.

bio

Jennie Nelson is a media post-graduate. An award-winning radio broadcaster and has been a footloose freelance writer since 2014.

She founded Off The Rocks in 2015; a health & wellness website dedicated to helping people overcome their struggles.

When she's not working, Jen can be found on the south coast of England. Lifting weights, making soup, drinking tea, reading books, watching films or barefoot on the beach. Mostly thinking about dinosaurs.

find out more:
website: www.offtherocks.co.uk
instagram: @off.the.rocks

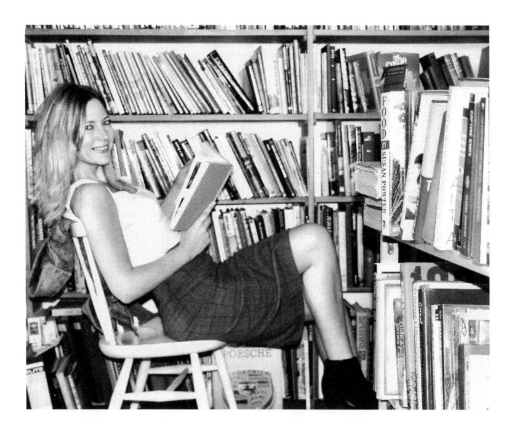

Printed in Great Britain
by Amazon